This report contains the collective views of an international group of experts and does not necessarily represent the decisions or the stated policy of the United Nations Environment Programme, the International Labour Organisation, or the World Health Organization.

Environmental Health Criteria 142

ALPHA-CYPERMETHRIN

First draft prepared by Dr E.A.H. van Heemstra-Lequin and Dr G.T. van Esch, Netherlands

Published under the joint sponsorship of the United Nations Environment Programme, the International Labour Organisation, and the World Health Organization

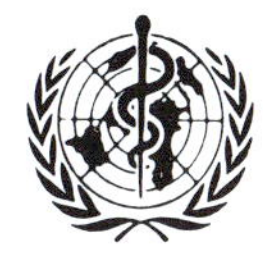

World Health Organization
Geneva, 1992

The **International Programme on Chemical Safety (IPCS)** is a joint venture of the United Nations Environment Programme, the International Labour Organisation, and the World Health Organization. The main objective of the IPCS is to carry out and disseminate evaluations of the effects of chemicals on human health and the quality of the environment. Supporting activities include the development of epidemiological, experimental laboratory, and risk-assessment methods that could produce internationally comparable results, and the development of manpower in the field of toxicology. Other activities carried out by the IPCS include the development of know-how for coping with chemical accidents, coordination of laboratory testing and epidemiological studies, and promotion of research on the mechanisms of the biological action of chemicals.

WHO Library Cataloguing in Publication Data

Alpha-cypermethrin.

(Environmental health criteria ; 142)

1.Environmental exposure 2.Pyrethrins - adverse effects
3.Pyrethrins - toxicity I.Series

ISBN 92 4 157142 X (NLM Classification: WA 240)
ISSN 0250-863X

Printed in Finland

92/9428 — Vammala — 5500

CONTENTS

ENVIRONMENTAL HEALTH CRITERIA FOR ALPHA-CYPERMETHRIN

WHO TASK GROUP ON ENVIRONMENTAL HEALTH CRITERIA FOR ALPHA-CYPERMETHRIN

Members

Dr V. Benes, Department of Toxicology and Reference Laboratory, Institute of Hygiene and Epidemiology, Prague, Czechoslovakia

Dr R. Drew, Key Centre for Toxicology, Department of Applied Biology, Royal Melbourne Institute for Technology, Melbourne, Australia (*Chairman*)

Dr S.K. Kashyap, National Institute of Occupational Health, Meghani Nagar, Ahmedabad, India

Dr J.I. Kundiev, Research Institute of Labour, Hygiene and Occupational Diseases, Ul. Saksaganskogo, Kiev, USSR (*Vice-Chairman*)

Dr K. Mitsumori, Division of Pathology, Biological Safety Research Center, National Institute of Hygienic Sciences, Setagaya-ku, Tokyo, Japan

Dr R.F. Shore, Ecotoxicology and Pollution Section, Institute of Terrestrial Ecology, Monks Wood Experimental Station, Abbots Ripton, Huntingdon, Cambridgeshire, United Kingdom

Dr G.J. van Esch, Bilthoven, Netherlands (*Joint Rapporteur*)

Dr E.A.H. van Heemstra-Lequin, Laren, Netherlands (*Joint Rapporteur*)

Dr S. Wong, Bureau of Chemical Hazards, Environmental Health Directorate, Department of National Health and Welfare, Tunney's Pasture, Ottawa, Ontario, Canada

Observers

Dr W.H. Gross, Fraunhofer Institute of Toxicology and Aerosol Research, Hanover, Germany

Dr J.R. Kielhorn, Fraunhofer Institute of Toxicology and Aerosol Research, Hanover, Germany

Dr C.M. Melber, Fraunhofer Institute of Toxicology and Aerosol Research, Hanover, Germany

Dr D.E. Owen, Shell Internationale Petroleum Maatschappij BV, The Hague, Netherlands

Secretariat

Dr R.F. Hertel, Fraunhofer Institute of Toxicology and Aerosol Research, Hanover, Germany

Dr K.W. Jager, International Programme on Chemical Safety, World Health Organization, Geneva, Switzerland (*Secretary*)

Mrs C. Partensky, Unit of Carcinogen Identification and Evaluation, International Agency for Research on Cancer, Lyon, France

NOTE TO READERS OF THE CRITERIA MONOGRAPHS

Every effort has been made to present information in the criteria monographs as accurately as possible without unduly delaying their publication. In the interest of all users of the Environmental Health Criteria monographs, readers are kindly requested to communicate any errors that may have occurred to the Director of the International Programme on Chemical Safety, World Health Organization, Geneva, Switzerland, in order that they may be included in corrigenda.

* * *

A detailed data profile and a legal file can be obtained from the International Register of Potentially Toxic Chemicals, Palais des Nations, 1211 Geneva 10, Switzerland (Telephone No. 7988400 or 7985850).

* * *

The proprietary information contained in this monograph cannot replace documentation for registration purposes, because the latter has to be closely linked to the source, the manufacturing route, and the purity/impurities of the substance to be registered. The data should be used in accordance with paragraphs 82-84 and recommendations paragraph 90 of the Second FAO Government Consultation (1982).

ENVIRONMENTAL HEALTH CRITERIA FOR ALPHA-CYPERMETHRIN

A WHO Task Group on Environmental Health Criteria for Alpha-cypermethrin met at the Fraunhofer Institute of Toxicology and Aerosol Research, Hanover, Germany, from 16 to 20 September 1990, and was sponsored by the German Ministry of the Environment. Dr R.F. Hertel welcomed the participants on behalf of the host institute. Dr K.W. Jager, IPCS, welcomed the participants on behalf of Dr M. Mercier, Director of the IPCS, and the three IPCS cooperating organizations (UNEP/ILO/WHO). The Group reviewed and revised the draft document and made an evaluation of the risks for human health and the environment from exposure to alpha-cypermethrin

The first draft was prepared by Dr E.A.H. van Heemstra-Lequin and Dr G.J. van Esch of the Netherlands. Dr van Esch prepared the second draft, incorporating the comments received following circulation of the first draft to the IPCS contact points for Environmental Health Criteria monographs.

Dr K.W. Jager and Dr P.G. Jenkins, both members of the IPCS Central Unit, were responsible for the technical development and editing, respectively.

The assistance of Shell in making available to the IPCS and the Task Group its proprietary toxicological information on alpha-cypermethrin is gratefully acknowledged. This allowed the Task Group to make its evaluation on the basis of more complete data.

* * *

Partial financial support for the publication of this monograph was kindly provided by the United States Department of Health and Human Services through a contract from the National Institute of Environmental Health Sciences, Research Triangle Park, North Carolina, USA - a WHO Collaborating Centre for Environmental Health Effects.

ABBREVIATIONS

CPA	cyclopropane carboxylic acid
EC	emulsifiable concentrate
EEC	European Economic Community
GC	gas chromatography
MRL	maximum residue level
MS	mass spectrophotometry
NOEL	no-observed-effect level
OECD	Organisation for Economic Co-operation and Development
OSC	oil-enhanced suspension concentrate
PBA	phenoxybenzoic acid
SC	suspension concentrate
ULV	ultra-low volume
WP	wettable powder

INTRODUCTION

Cypermethrin (alpha-cyano-3-phenoxybenzyl-3-(2,2-dichlorovinyl)-2,2-dimethylcyclopropanecarboxylate) is a racemic mixture of eight isomers. These eight isomers consist of two groups, those with a cis orientation across the cyclopropyl ring of the dichlorovinyl and ester groups and those with a trans orientation.

Alpha-cypermethrin is a mixture of two of the four cis isomers present to approximately 25% in cypermethrin, i.e. the (1R, cis)S and the (1S, cis)R isomers. The structure of the eight isomers is summarized in Fig. 1.

In this monograph the toxicological information specifically related to alpha-cypermethrin is summarized and compared with the data on cypermethrin. An evaluation of the full data on cypermethrin, which is also relevant for alpha-cypermethrin, is given in Environmental Health Criteria 82: Cypermethrin (WHO, 1989). The summary, evaluation, conclusions and recommendations of that monograph are added here as Appendix I.

1. SUMMARY AND EVALUATION; CONCLUSIONS AND RECOMMENDATIONS

1.1 Summary and evaluation

1.1.1 Identity, use, environmental fate and environmental levels

Alpha-cypermethrin contains more than 90% of the insecticidally most active enantiomer pair of the four cis isomers of cypermethrin as a racemic mixture.

It is a highly active pyrethroid insecticide, effective against a wide range of pests encountered in agriculture and animal husbandry. It is supplied as emulsifiable concentrate, ultra-low-volume formulation, suspension concentrate and in mixtures with other insecticides.

The technical product is a crystalline powder with good solubility in acetone, cyclohexanone and xylene, but its solubility in water is low. It is stable under acidic and neutral conditions but hydrolyses at pH 12-13. It decomposes above 220 °C.

No information on levels of alpha-cypermethrin in air is available.

In water, alpha-cypermethrin is likely to be degraded by photochemical and biological processes. Surface and sub-surface water in a pond oversprayed with 15 g/ha active ingredient contained 5% and 19% of the applied dose one day after spraying and 0.1% and 2% of the applied dose seven days later. About 5% of the applied dose was present in sediment 16 days after application.

Alpha-cypermethrin is likely to be absorbed strongly onto soil particles. Residues in soil were below 0.1 mg/kg one year after treatment with 0.5 kg active ingredient per ha.

The *n*-octanol/water partition coefficient of alpha-cypermethrin is 1.4×10^5 ($\log P_{ow} = 5.16$).

The recommended application rates of alpha-cypermethrin are lower than those of cypermethrin because the former is biologically more active. As a result, residues on crops are low, and following the use of recommended application rates the residues in crops are between 0.05 and 1 mg/kg. Residues in marine catfish treated at between 0.001 and 0.05% w/w active ingredient were 0.3-30 mg/kg one week after storage and 0.22-4.0 mg/kg after 15 weeks of storage.

1.1.2 Kinetics and metabolism

Alpha-cypermethrin administered orally to rats is eliminated, in the urine, as the sulfate conjugate of 3-(4-hydroxyphenoxy) benzoic acid and, in the faeces, partly as unchanged compound. Approximately 90% of a single oral dose is eliminated from the body over a 4-day period, 78% within the first day. Residues in tissues are low except in fat tissue. The concentration in fat 3 days after a single oral dose of 2 mg/kg was 0.4 mg/kg. Elimination from the fat is biphasic; the half-life for the initial phase is 2.5 days and for the second phase 17-26 days.

Alpha-cypermethrin is metabolized by cleavage of its ester bond. In the rat, the phenoxybenzyl alcohol portion of the molecule is hydroxylated and conjugated with sulfate; the cyclopropane carboxylic acid portion is also conjugated (probably as a glucuronide) prior to urinary excretion. Studies with liver microsomes from rats, rabbits and man have demonstrated that esteric hydrolysis and oxidative pathways can occur in all three species but esteric hydrolysis is the more prominent pathway for liver preparations from rabbit and man.

In humans, 43% of an oral dose (0.25-0.75 mg) was excreted within 24 h in the urine as free or conjugated *cis*-cyclopropane carboxylic acid. The urinary excretion was not increased after five successive daily doses.

High concentrations (up to 1156 mg/kg) of alpha-cypermethrin were found in the wool of sheep 14 days after the application of a dip or pour-on formulation. Low levels were found in subcutaneous fat (up to 0.04 mg/kg). After treating calves along the mid-dorsal line with 10 ml of a 1.6% formulation, no alpha-cypermethrin was found in muscle and liver. The maximum concentration in perirenal fat over a 14-day period was 0.26 mg/kg.

After treating lactating cows along the mid-dorsal line with up to 0.2 g active ingredient, alpha-cypermethrin residues of 0.003 to 0.005 mg/litre were found in the milk from 3 out of 15 treated animals.

1.1.3 Effects on laboratory mammals and in vitro *test systems*

Alpha-cypermethrin has moderate to high acute oral toxicity to rodents. The LD_{50} values in mice and rats are highly variable and depend on the concentration of the compound and vehicle. For practical purposes an LD_{50} value of 80 mg/kg body weight is considered representative. However, some reported acute oral LD_{50} values are higher. Acute oral exposure results in clinical signs associated with central nervous system activity.

Single dermal applications of alpha-cypermethrin to mice and rats at 100 and 500 mg/kg body weight, respectively, did not cause mortality or signs of intoxication. Similarly, a 4-h inhalation exposure of rats to an atmospheric concentration of 400 mg/m^3 did not result in mortality or clinical signs.

Technical alpha-cypermethrin has been reported to be minimally irritating to rabbit skin. Some alpha-cypermethrin formulations cause severe eye irritation. Technical alpha-cypermethrin is not a skin sensitizer. In guinea-pigs, alpha-cypermethrin caused stimulation of sensory nerve-endings in the skin.

Short-term exposure of rats to alpha-cypermethrin at concentrations up to 200 mg/kg diet per day for 5 weeks or up to 180 mg/kg diet per day for 13 weeks did not cause toxic effects. At higher dose levels, rats exhibited signs of intoxication associated with pathology of the nervous system, decreased growth, or increased liver and kidney weights. No clear haematological, clinical chemistry or histopathological effects were evident.

In a 13-week oral dog study, the highest dose of 270 mg/kg diet caused signs of intoxication, but all other parameters examined (including haematology, clinical chemistry, urinalysis, organ weights, gross pathology and histopathology) were unaffected. The no-observed-effect level (NOEL) was 90 mg/kg diet (equivalent to 2.25 mg/kg body weight per day).

An oral study in rats demonstrated that alpha-cypermethrin induces neurotoxicity due to histopathological alterations of the tibial and sciatic nerves, axonal degeneration and increased beta-galactosidase activity.

No data are available on long-term toxicity, reproductive toxicity, teratogenicity or immunotoxicity.

From the available data on alpha-cypermethrin, it can be concluded that this compound is non-mutagenic in tests with *Salmonella typhimurium*, *Escherichia coli* and *Saccharomyces cerevisiae*, and *in vivo* and *in vitro* tests with rat liver cells for the induction of chromosome aberration and production of DNA single-strand damage. No increase in chromosomal aberrations was seen in rat bone marrow cells.

No data are available on the carcinogenicity of alpha-cypermethrin.

1.1.4 Effects on humans

Exposure of the general population to alpha-cypermethrin is negligible, provided its use follows good agricultural practice. Occupational dermal exposure in operators during mixing/loading, during spraying and washing of the equipment was found to be up to 2.94 mg, 0.61 mg and 0.73 mg, respectively.

In a study of exposure to alpha-cypermethrin during formulation, exposure levels were assessed by personal and static monitoring of atmospheric concentrations and measurement of urinary alpha-cypermethrin metabolites. The group mean personal exposure levels on the two days while formulating technical concentrates were 2.8 and 4.9 mg/m^3, whereas the group mean personal exposure to technical material on day 3 was 54.1 mg/m^3. No metabolites could be detected in urine (limit of detection, 0.02 mg/litre). During formulation, skin sensations were reported but these were only mild.

No poisoning incidents have been reported.

1.1.5 Effects on other organisms in the laboratory and field

The 48 and 96-h EC_{50} (growth) value for the freshwater alga *Selenastrum capricornutum* is above 100 μg/litre.

Alpha-cypermethrin is highly toxic to aquatic invertebrates. The 24- and 48-h EC_{50} (immobilization) values for *Daphnia magna* are 1.0 and 0.3 μg/litre, respectively, and the 24-h LC_{50} value for *Gammarus pulex* is 0.05 μg/litre. Alpha-cypermethrin is highly toxic to a number of aquatic arthropod taxa, but is of lower toxicity to molluscs. The short-term toxicity of the compound can be reduced by formulation of the product as an oil-enhanced suspension. Although spray drift may result in toxic effects on aquatic invertebrates, the rapid loss of alpha-cypermethrin from the water gives potential for recovery.

Alpha-cypermethrin is highly toxic to fish. The 96-h LC_{50} values range between 0.7 and 350 μg/litre depending upon the formulation. Emulsifiable concentrate formulations are much more toxic than suspension concentrate, wettable powder and micro-encapsulated formulations. The hazard of alpha-cypermethrin to aquatic invertebrates and fish lies in its acute toxicity. There is no evidence for the occurrence of cumulative effects as a result of long-term exposure.

No data are available concerning the effects of alpha-cypermethrin on soil microbes. Sewage bacteria were not affected by a concentration of 3 mg/litre in a closed system.

The toxicity of alpha-cypermethrin to certain Carabid beetles and neuropteran larvae is relatively low, and there is limited hazard to pre-adult stages of parasitoid Hymenoptera. Small-plot and large-scale field studies have demonstrated a low hazard of alpha-cypermethrin to Carabid and Staphylinid beetles but a relatively high hazard to Linyphiid spiders. The effects on populations were limited to a single growing season. Furthermore, alpha-cypermethrin has a low hazard to Syrphid larvae but has a significant effect on Coccinellids. However, the rapid dissipation of the residues on foliage gives the potential for these animals to recolonize rapidly.

Field application of alpha-cypermethrin had no adverse effects on the relative abundance of entomophages within the arthropod communities. Its use in small grain cereals would not be associated with pest "resurgence" or the development of secondary pest infestations.

In laboratory tests, the toxicity of alpha-cypermethrin to earthworms is low. No mortality was recorded after 14 days for worms exposed to up to 100 mg/kg of artificial soil.

In laboratory acute toxicity tests, alpha-cypermethrin was found to be highly toxic to bees. Oral administration of an emulsifiable concentrate formulation gave a 24-h LD_{50} of 0.13 μg/bee, whereas the corresponding value for topical administration was 0.03 μg/bee (technical product) or 0.11 μg/bee (EC). The high toxicity of alpha-cypermethrin to bees did not manifest itself in field trials, probably as a result of the short-lived repellent effect of alpha-cypermethrin which causes a decline in bee foraging behaviour and, thus, in exposure.

No data for the toxicity of alpha-cypermethrin to birds are available.

1.2 Conclusions

1.2.1 General population

When applied according to good agricultural practice, exposure of the general population to alpha-cypermethrin is low and is unlikely to present a hazard.

1.2.2 Occupational exposure

With good work practices, hygiene measures, and safety precautions, the use of alpha-cypermethrin is unlikely to present a hazard to those occupationally exposed to it. The occurrence of "facial sensations" is an indication of exposure. Under these circumstances work practices should be reviewed.

1.2.3 Environment

With recommended application rates, it is unlikely that alpha-cypermethrin will attain levels of environmental significance. It is highly toxic to aquatic arthropods, fish and honey-bees under laboratory conditions. Significant toxic effects on non-target invertebrates and fish are only likely to occur in cases of spillage, overspraying and misuse.

1.3 Recommendations

- Contamination of surface waters with alpha-cypermethrin should be avoided.
- Alpha-cypermethrin binds strongly to particles. Further ecotoxicological studies on the effects of alpha-cypermethrin on sediment-dwelling organisms should be carried out, since this subject seems to have received little attention.
- The gastrointestinal absorption of alpha-cypermethrin should be investigated under various conditions.
- The fate of dermally applied alpha-cypermethrin should be investigated.

- Further information on the long-term toxicity/carcinogenicity and immunotoxicity of alpha-cypermethrin should be obtained.

2. IDENTITY, PHYSICAL AND CHEMICAL PROPERTIES, AND ANALYTICAL METHODS

2.1 Identity

2.1.1 Primary constituent

Chemical structure:	racemic mixture of the two stereoisomers indicated by boxes in Fig. 1
Empirical formula:	$C_{22}H_{19}NO_3Cl_2$
Relative molecular mass:	416.3
Chemical name: (IUPAC)	a racemate comprising (S)-alpha-cyano-3-phenoxybenzyl (1R,3R)-3-(2,2-dichloro-vinyl)-2,2-dimethylcyclopropanecarboxylate and (R)-alpha-cyano-3-phenoxybenzyl (1S,3S)-3-(2,2-dichlorovinyl)-2,2-dimethylcyclopropanecarboxylate; a racemate comprising (S)-alpha-cyano-3-phenoxybenzyl (1R)-*cis*-3(2,2-dichloro-vinyl)-2,2-dimethylcyclopropanecarboxylate and (R)-alpha-cyano-3-phenoxybenzyl (1S)-*cis*-3-(2,2-dichlorovinyl)-2,2-dimethylcyclopropanecarboxylate
(Chemical Abstracts)	[1alpha(S*),3alpha}-(±)-cyano(3-phenoxyphenyl)methyl 3-(2,2-dichloroethenyl)-2,2-dimethylcyclopropanecarboxylate (9CI) (From: Worthing & Hance, 1991)
Common name:	alpha-cypermethrin (alphamethrin and alfoxylate are non-official names)
Code numbers:	WL 85 871; OMS 3004
CAS registry number:	[67375-30-8] correct stereochemistry; [52315-07-8] (formerly [69865-74-0], [86752-99-0], [86753-92-6] cypermethrin (no stereochemistry stated) were sometimes used in Chemical Abstracts)

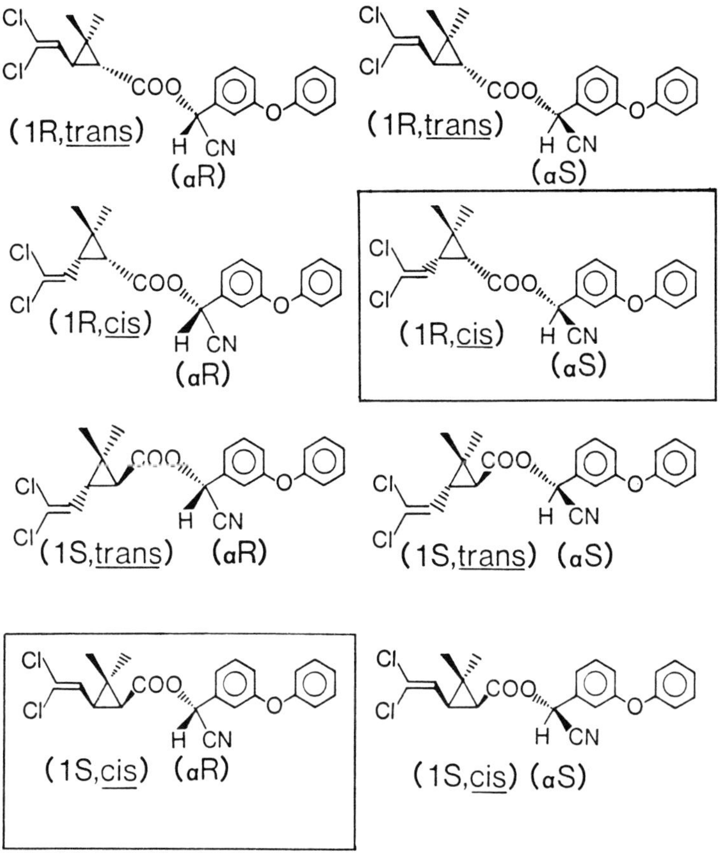

Fig. 1. Chemical structures of eight stereoisomers. Alpha-cypermethrin comprises the two framed structures.

2.1.2 Technical product

Common trade names: Fastac, Concord, Fendona, Renegade

Purity: technical grade: > 90% pure (m/m)

Impurities: no data.

2.2 Physical and chemical properties

Alpha-cypermethrin is a racemic mixture of the two stereoisomers (1:1) indicated by boxes in Fig. 1 and is a crystalline powder. Some physical and chemical properties of alpha-cypermethrin are given in Table 1.

Table 1. Physical and chemical properties of alpha-cypermethrin (pure enantiomeric pair; purity > 99%)

Boiling point	200 °C at 9.3 N/m^2
Melting point	80.5 °C
Vapour pressure (20 °C)	170 nPa (1.7 x 10^7 N/m^2)
Density	1.12 g/cm^3 at 20 °C 1.28 g/cm^3 at 22 °C
Solubility (25 °C)	0.005-0.01 mg/litre water; 620 g/litre acetone; 515 g/litre cyclohexanone; 7 g/kg hexane; 351 g/litre xylene
Stability	It is stable under acidic or neutral conditions (pH 3-7) but hydrolyses in strongly alkaline media (pH 12-13). It decomposes above 220 °C. Field data indicate that in practice it is stable to air and light.
Partition coefficient *n*-octanol/water	log P_{ow} 5.16 (P_{ow} = 1.4 x 10^5)

From: Langner (1980); Shell (1983a); Worthing & Hance (1991).

The water solubility of alpha-cypermethrin (98.0%), calculated as the sum of the cis-1 and the cis-2 isomer (ratio 2.6:97.4) concentrations, at 20 °C in 0.01 M buffers at pH values of approximately 4 to 9, ranges from 4.59 to 7.87 μg/litre, as measured by the OECD and EEC microcolumn techniques. In distilled water alone the solubility is slightly less, i.e. 2.06 μg/litre. The solubility is not strongly dependent on pH values within the range of 4 to 9. It is likely that ionic strength differences account for differences in solubility between values in pure water and in the buffer solutions (Baldwin, 1990).

2.3 Formulations

The following formulations exist:

- "Fastac", EC (20-100 g/litre), WP (50 g/kg), SC (15-250 g/litre), ULV (6 to 15 g/litre);
- "Fendona" and "Renegade", EC (50 or 100 g/litre), SC (250 g/litre), WP (50 g/kg).

Combination with other active ingredients also exist, e.g., "Azofas" (alpha-cypermethrin and monocrotophos) and combinations of alpha-cypermethrin with methomyl or Fenobucarb (Worthing & Hance, 1991).

2.4 Conversion factors

1 ppm = 17.02 mg/m^3
1 mg/m^3 - 0.059 ppm

2.5 Analytical methods

2.5.1 Sampling

2.5.1.1 Air

Samples are collected by drawing a measured volume of air through a 37-mm diameter silver membrane filter with a glass fibre pre-filter. They are analysed for total pyrethroid content (*cis-* and *trans-*cypermethrin isomers) by gas chromatography with electron capture detection (ECD). The limit of determination is 0.01 μg/filter (see Table 2) (Armitage, 1984).

2.5.1.2 Surface-wipe

Surface-wipe samples are collected using a filter paper wetted with diethyl ether. These samples are analysed for total pyrethroid content (*cis-* and *trans-*cypermethrin isomers) by gas chromatography with flame ionization detection (FID). The limit of determination is 0.03 mg/filter (see Table 2) (Armitage, 1984).

2.5.2 Methods for determination

A method for the determination of alpha-cypermethrin in technical material and formulated products, excluding suspension concentrates, was described by Shell (1987a). This method is also used to determine the ratio of the enantiomer pairs cis 1 to cis 2.

Table 2. Analytical methods for alpha-cypermethrin in air, soil, water and biological media[a]

Sample	Extraction	Clean-up	Detection and quantification	Recovery	Limit of determination	References
Air	20% ethyl acetate in hexane	column chromatography chromosorb W.HP.	gas chromatography with electron capture detection	-	0.01 µg/filter	Armitage (1984)
Surface wipe	20% ethyl acetate in hexane	column chromatography chromosorb W.HP.	gas chromatography with flame ionization detection	-	30 µg/filter	Armitage (1984)
Soil	anhydrous sodium sulfate with acetone/hexane	liquid-solid chromatography using Florisil	packed column gas chromatography, electron capture detection; confirmation by capillary GC and packed column GC-MS	95-100%[b]	10 µg/kg	Shell (1990b)
Water	solvent partition with hexane	Florisil disposable cartridge	capillary gas-liquid chromatography, electron-capture detection; confirmation by GC-MS	80-100%[c]	0.01 µg/litre	Shell (1990a)
Crops	anhydrous sodium sulfate with acetone/hexane	partition between hexane and water/acetonitrile; liquid-solid chromatography using Florisil	packed column gas chromatography, electron capture detection; confirmation by capillary GC and packed column GC-MS	90-100%[b]	10 µg/kg	Shell (1989a)

Table 2 (contd).

Animal tissues	acetone/hexane mixture	partition with acetonitrile or hexane-acetonitrile; liquid-solid chromatography on Florisil	gas-liquid chromatography, electron capture detection; confirmation by GC-MS	80-100%[d]	10 μg/kg	Shell (1988a)
Milk	diethyl ether/hexane; Extrelut extraction column	cyano Bond Elut cartridge	gas-liquid chromatography, electron capture detection; confirmation by GC-MS	90-100%[e]	1 μg/litre	Shell (1988b)
Blood (rat)	acetone	partition with hexane (washed with water); dried with sodium sulfate; liquid-solid chromatography on Florisil	packed column gas chromatography, electron capture detection; confirmation by capillary GC and GC-MS	-	10 μg/litre	Shell (1986)

[a] Details of the analytical methods are available from Shell International Chemical Company, London. These methods differentiate between alpha-cypermethrin and the other isomers.
[b] Over the concentration range 0.05-0.5 mg/kg
[c] Over the concentration range 0.05-0.5 μg/litre
[d] Concentrations 0.1-0.2 mg/kg
[e] Over the concentration range 0.005-0.02 mg/litre

The alpha-cypermethrin content is determined by means of high-performance liquid chromatography (HPLC), using a column packed with Zorbax SIL, together with ultraviolet detection at 230 nm (Shell, 1987a).

Methods have been described for the determination of alpha-cypermethrin in water, soil, crops, and animal tissues and fluids (see Table 2).

3. SOURCES OF HUMAN AND ENVIRONMENTAL EXPOSURE

3.1 Natural occurrence

Alpha-cypermethrin does not occur in nature.

3.2 Anthropogenic sources

3.2.1 Production levels and processes

Alpha-cypermethrin is manufactured from *cis*-2,2,dimethyl-3-(2",2"-dichlorovinyl)-cyclopropane carboxylate (*cis*-DVO), 3-phenoxy benzaldehyde (POAL) and sodium cyanide.

After removal of the solvent, the *cis*-cypermethrin is epimerized into alpha-cypermethrin. Solid alpha-cypermethrin crystals separate and are filtered, washed and dried under vacuum before drumming-off[1].

No data are available on production levels.

3.2.2 Use

Alpha-cypermethrin has been available commercially since late 1983. It is a potent insecticide effective against a wide range of pests, particularly *Lepidoptera* and *Coleoptera* in citrus, cotton, forestry, fruit, rice, soybeans, tomatoes, vegetables, grapes and other crops, at a concentration of 5-30 g active ingredient per ha. Good control of plant-sucking *Hemiptera* can also be obtained if the insecticide is applied before populations have become established. It also controls soil-dwelling *Lepidoptera.*

Alpha-cypermethrin can be used in most crops for either curative or preventive treatment. It can replace conventional insecticides in short-interval spray programmes, or the longer residual performance may be exploited to reduce the number of sprays per season. Either option may be chosen since no reports of phytotoxicity have been received even when sensitive crops have been involved in repeated applications. It controls

---

1 Manufacturing process of alpha-cypermethrin; Shell International Chemical Company; letter dated 10 January 1989 (ref. CTMAR/4)

ectoparasites (*Boophilus microplus* at a concentration of 50 mg/litre), including strains resistant to organophosphorus pesticides, as well as sheep lice and *Melophagus ovinus*.

Rapid knockdown and residual control of biting flies in and around animal housing have been obtained following direct spray application to animals or structural surfaces. Furthermore, alpha-cypermethrin controls *Blattellidae*, *Culicidae*, flies and other nuisance or disease-carrying insects, at a level of 10-30 mg/m^2, with good persistence on most surfaces (Fisher et al., 1983; Worthing & Hance, 1991).

Alpha-cypermethrin is available as an emulsifiable concentrate, ultra-low-volume formulation and suspension concentrate (flowable formulations). Mixtures with organophosphorus and carbamate insecticides have also been developed. Details of formulations are given in section 2.3.

4. ENVIRONMENTAL TRANSPORT, DISTRIBUTION AND TRANSFORMATION

4.1 Transport and distribution between media

Data relevant to alpha-cypermethrin can be found in Environmental Health Criteria 82: Cypermethrin (WHO, 1989).

4.1.1 Air

No information on the transport of alpha-cypermethrin in air is available, but its volatility is very low.

4.1.2 Water

Alpha-cypermethrin as an emulsifiable concentrate (EC) was sprayed from the air (15 g active ingredient/ha) to a field along one side of which ran a freshwater ditch. The fate and biological effects of spray drift in the ditch were monitored for 7 weeks after the application (see sections 9.2.1.2 and 9.2.2.2). Deposition on the surface of the ditch was around 5 g active ingredient/ha (30% of the nominal application rate). Alpha-cypermethrin concentrations in the sub-surface water were 0.6 μg/litre shortly after the application and decreased to < 0.02 μg/litre within 2 to 4 days. No contamination of the water was found 200 m beyond either end of the treated field (Garforth & Woodbridge, 1984).

Two freshwater ponds were treated with an EC formulation of alpha-cypermethrin in 1987. One pond was oversprayed with 15 g active ingredient/ha, while the other was treated with the same amount of alpha-cypermethrin but by direct incorporation into the water. A third pond served as a control. One day after the treatment, 5% of the applied substance was found in the surface film of the oversprayed pond and 19% in the sub-surface water. Residue levels in both compartments subsequently declined rapidly so that one week later only 0.1 and 2% were still present, respectively. In the pond that received direct treatment, 37% of the applied alpha-cypermethrin was found in the sub-surface water one day after treatment. The concentration subsequently declined more rapidly than in the oversprayed pond so that one week later only 2% was present. The concentration of alpha-cypermethrin found in the sediment samples from both ponds 16 days after treatment indicated that approximately 5% of the alpha-cypermethrin applied was present at that time. Thereafter the concentration decreased and was less than 3% in the sediment 33 days after application. In a bioassay test, the water in both ponds was found to be acutely toxic to *Gammarus pulex* for at least 4 days after application. After a further 29 days, the water was no longer acutely toxic. The sediment was not toxic to *Gammarus pulex* (Pearson, 1990).

4.1.3 Soil

A trial in the United Kingdom (Reculver) investigated the decay of alpha-cypermethrin in sandy-clay soil treated with a diluted EC formulation at a dosage rate of 0.5 kg active ingredient per ha. Samples of soil were taken from the 0-15 cm layer of each plot at various intervals over a period of one year. Once a year a sample was also taken from the 15-30 cm layer. The residue immediately after the application was 0.07 mg/kg soil in the 0-15 cm layer, and within 2 weeks this had declined by 50%. The residues of alpha-cypermethrin in samples from the 0-15 cm layer and 15-30 cm layer taken 40 weeks and 52 weeks after application were below the limit of determination, i.e. 0.01 mg/kg (Forbes & Knight, 1983).

After one year, a second application to the bare soil was made and again a diluted EC formulation was applied at a dosage rate of 0.5 kg active ingredient/ha. Samples were taken at various intervals during this second year. Residues of alpha-cypermethrin in the 0-15 cm soil layer declined from 0.19 mg/kg immediately after treatment to 0.11 mg/kg after 2.1 weeks and < 0.01 mg/kg after 49 weeks. In samples from the 15-30 cm layer no residues (< 0.01 mg/kg) were detectable 23 and 49 weeks after application (Forbes & Burden, 1984). In the third year of the trial, another application to the same plots was made with the EC formulation at a dosage rate of 0.5 kg active ingredient/ha. Residues of alpha-cypermethrin in the 0-15 cm layer declined from 0.20 mg/kg immediately after treatment to 0.08 mg/kg after 18 weeks and 0.01 mg/kg after 52 weeks. Residues were not detectable in the 15-30 cm layer sampled after 32 and 52 weeks. Over the three years of the trial there was no indication of a build-up of alpha-cypermethrin residues in the surface soil layer or any evidence to suggest leaching of the compound into sub-surface soil layers (Forbes & Wales, 1985a).

A further trial was carried out in the United Kingdom (Coates) to study the decay of alpha-cypermethrin applied to a peat type soil as a diluted EC formulation at a dosage rate of 0.5 kg active ingredient/ha. As in the Reculver study, residues were determined in the 0-15 cm layer at various intervals and in the 15-30 cm layer 32 weeks after application. At the beginning of the second and third year, one application was made as at the beginning of the first year. The residue in the 0-15 cm layer immediately after the first application was 0.65 mg/kg declining to 0.36 mg/kg within 2 weeks and to 0.30 mg/kg after 8 weeks. After 16 weeks, the residue was 0.05 mg/kg or less. In the 15-30 cm layer, no residues were found after 32 weeks (Forbes & Mackay, 1983). Immediately after the second application, the residue in the 0-15 cm layer was 0.65 mg/kg; after two weeks the level was 0.36 mg/kg and declined to 0.07 mg/kg by 48 weeks after application. No residues were found in the 15-30 cm layer (Forbes & Wales, 1985b).

In the third year, a residue level of 0.55 mg/kg was found in the 0-15 cm layer immediately after treatment, declining to 0.20 mg/kg within 8 weeks and to 0.09 mg/kg after 50 weeks. In the 15-30 cm layer, residues of 0.01 and 0.03 mg/kg were found after 40 and 50 weeks respectively. In this 3-year trial there was no indication of a build-up of alpha-cypermethrin residues in the surface soil layers, or any evidence to suggest significant leaching into sub-surface soil layers (Coveney & Forbes, 1986).

4.2 Biotransformation

4.2.1 Biodegradation

Alpha-cypermethrin has been tested for "ready biodegradability" in two tests: a) the closed bottle and modified Sturm test, and b) growth inhibition in a *Pseudomonas fluorescens* growth test. In these tests, mineralization of alpha-cypermethrin was not detected. It was not degraded in these two tests and hence is not considered to be readily biodegradable (Stone & Watkinson, 1983).

Maloney et al. (1988) studied the microbial transformation of technical alpha-cypermethrin (96.3% pure) in aerobic batch enrichment cultures. These microbial enrichments, which contained *Pseudomonas fluorescens* (SM-1), *Achromobacter* sp. and *Bacillus cereus*, were able to transform alpha-cypermethrin with a half-life of 7 to 14 days at a concentration of 50 mg/litre in the presence of 0.05% Tween 80 (v/v). One of the major transformation products was 3-phenoxybenzoic acid, which was further transformed to 4-hydroxy-3-phenoxybenzoic acid.

McMinn (1983a) investigated the degradation under aerobic conditions of alpha-cypermethrin, labelled with ^{14}C in the benzyl ring, in two types of soil, i.e. sandy clay loam and clay loam. The soils were treated with 1 mg of the labelled material and gently agitated to distribute the insecticide. Soils samples were removed for analysis 2.5, 6, 10, 20 and 42 weeks after treatment. The initial degradation half-lives were 27 and 13 weeks for sandy clay loam and clay loam, respectively. However, after 42 weeks the percentage of applied radioactivity remaining unchanged was 28.9 and 21.6%, respectively, for the two soils. The formation of total organo-soluble products after 42 weeks was 32.2 and 24.3% for sandy clay loam and clay loam, respectively. Total extractable and total non-extractable radioactivity for sandy clay loam was 32.5 and 18.0% and for clay loam 25.3 and 32.0%, respectively. Metabolites were found in both cases at levels of 2 to 3%. Unchanged alpha-cypermethrin was present, and the degradation products had similar chromatographic mobilities to the previously identified major products of cypermethrin (McMinn, 1983b).

4.2.2 Bioaccumulation

The *n*-octanol/water partition coefficient of alpha-cypermethrin is 1.4×10^5 (log $P_{ow} = 5.16$), compared to a value for cypermethrin of 2×10^6 (log $P_{ow} = 6.3$). The actual bioaccumulation in fish found experimentally for cypermethrin is lower than might be expected from the partition coefficient. This should also apply to alpha-cypermethrin, because the pathway and rate of metabolism are comparable with those of cypermethrin (Shell, 1983b; WHO, 1989).

5. ENVIRONMENTAL LEVELS AND HUMAN EXPOSURE

5.1 Environmental levels

Information relevant to alpha-cypermethrin was given in Environmental Health Criteria 82: Cypermethrin (WHO, 1989).

5.1.1 Soil

In a study on the deposition of alpha-cypermethrin on the orchard floor following commercial application to apple trees, alpha-cypermethrin (100 g EC/litre) was applied at a nominal dose rate of 26 g/ha using a tractor-driven "Kinkelder" mist-blower. Following normal practice, spray runs were made between each row of trees and then around the perimeter of the orchard. One hour after spraying, pesticide deposits were collected in foil-lined trays positioned on the orchard floor and analysed. Deposition was found to be variable, ranging from 10 to 76% of the nominal application rate (Hillaby, 1988).

5.2 Food

5.2.1 Crops

Residue data on cypermethrin have been evaluated by the Joint FAO/WHO Meeting on Pesticide Residues (FAO/WHO, 1980, 1982).

Alpha-cypermethrin application rates to crops range from 5 to 30 g active ingredient/ha. Residue data have been obtained from supervised trials in many countries. The residue concentrations of alpha-cypermethrin derived from recommended application rates vary from 0.05 to 1.0 mg/kg product (Shell, 1984).

A study was carried out to determine whether there was significant isomerization of alpha-cypermethrin after treatment of certain crops. Grapes were treated with 10% EC applied at a rate of 18 g active ingredient/ha, and apples and lettuce with 10% EC at 15 g active ingredient/ha. Samples were taken 3 and 7 days (grapes), 7 days (apples) and 10 days (lettuce) after treatment. Residues of 0.17 and 0.09 mg/kg were found on grapes, 0.05 mg/kg on apples and 0.17 mg/kg on lettuce, but none of the samples showed any significant isomer conversion of alpha-cypermethrin (Bosio, 1982).

In 1983 two trials were carried out in Canada in which alpha-cypermethrin was applied with a knapsack sprayer to maize (sweetcorn). Five applications with diluted 10% EC formulations at a dosage rate of 20 g active ingredient/ha were made, samples were harvested 7 days after the last application, and the husks, grain and cobs were analysed separately. Alpha-cypermethrin residues of 0.38 mg/kg were found in the husks, but no residues (limit of determination, 0.01 mg/kg) were found in the grain or the cobs (Forbes & Cole, 1986).

5.2.2 *Fish*

To reduce blow-fly infestations during the curing of marine catfish, the fish were dipped in EC solutions (15 g/litre) at various concentrations (0.001-0.05% active ingredient w/v) between the salting and drying stages of the curing process. Dipping after the salting stage in a 0.001% solution of the EC proved to be effective. The levels of residues in treated fish were dependent on the season (wet and dry season), storage time, concentration of the dip solution and the size of the fish. In the wet season, the range was from 0.9 to 2.8 mg/kg, whereas in the dry season it was from 0.26 to 30.0 after one week of storage and 0.22 to 4.0 mg/kg (wet weight of homogenized fish) after 15 weeks of storage (Forbes, 1985).

5.2.3 *Milk*

A trial was carried out in 1987 in the United Kingdom where lactating cows were treated with pour-on formulations of alpha-cypermethrin. Two formulations were used containing either 10 g/litre or 15 g/litre (see also section 6.1.2). Either 10 ml or 20 ml of formulation containing 0.1, 0.15 or 0.2 g active ingredient was applied along the mid-dorsal line of five cows for each treatment. Milk samples were taken 1, 2, 3, 4, 7, 14 and 21 days after treatment for the analysis of alpha-cypermethrin. The residues of alpha-cypermethrin in milk were at a maximum from 2 to 4 days after treatment. Generally, residues were highest in the 0.2 g group, the maximum concentration being 0.005 mg/litre (in two samples only). By day 21 the residues in the milk from all treated cows were < 0.002 mg/litre (the limit of determination) (Sherren, 1988b).

5.3 Human exposure

In a study to quantify the maximum potential dermal exposure of operators to crop protection products, 13 exposure pads were mounted on each of three operators and chemicals adhering to gloves were analysed. The operation involved three distinct stages: mixing product and loading the tractor; spraying; and washing-up the equipment and tractor after the exercise. The total dermal exposure for the three operators was: mixing/loading, 2.45, 0.57 and 2.94 mg/operation; spraying, 0.38, 0.61 and 0.40 mg/h; and washing-up, 0.12, 0.29 and 0.73 mg/operation (Senior & Lavers, 1990a,b).

6. KINETICS AND METABOLISM

Both cis and trans isomers of cypermethrin are metabolized via cleavage of the ester bond to phenoxybenzoic acid (PBA) and cyclopropane carboxylic acid (CPA). The PBA moiety is mainly excreted as a conjugate. The type of conjugate differs in a number of animal species. PBA is further metabolized to a hydroxy derivative and conjugated as a glucuronate or sulfate. The CPA moiety is mainly excreted as a glucuronate. Consistent with the lipophilic nature of cypermethrin, the highest tissue concentrations are found in body fat, skin, liver, kidneys, adrenals and ovaries. The elimination from fat is approximately 3 to 4 times slower for the cis isomers than for the trans isomers (WHO, 1989).

6.1 Absorption, elimination, retention and turnover

6.1.1 Rats

Alpha-cypermethrin labelled in the ^{14}C-benzyl moiety has been studied in Wistar rats at a concentration of approximately 2 mg/kg body weight in corn oil. The compound, which was given by stomach tube, was rapidly broken down and the radioactivity was mainly eliminated in the urine as the sulfate conjugate of 3-(4-hydroxyphenoxy)benzoic acid (40-45% of the dose). Approximately 35% of the dose was eliminated in the faeces, 20% of which was unchanged alpha-cypermethrin. The proportion of the dose excreted in the urine and faeces within the first 24 h was approximately 78% and within 4 days was 90%. Residues in major organs and tissues of rats 4 days after a single oral dose were in general low: liver, 0.03 and 0.05; skin, 0.04 and 0.02; adrenals, 0.03 and 0.06; and kidneys, 0.02 and 0.02 (values are expressed as mg equivalent of alpha-cypermethrin/kg tissue for females and males, respectively). However, in body fat, higher residues were found (0.22 and 0.42 mg/kg). The release from skin and fat was biphasic in nature. The half-life of elimination of radioactivity from fat was approximately 2.5 days for the initial phase and 17-26 days for the slower phase (the half-life of elimination from fat for *cis*-cypermethrin was 18.9 days). The half-life values for skin were 2 days for the initial phase and 40 days for the slower phase. The radioactivity in liver and kidneys was eliminated apparently by a monophasic process. More than 95% of the residue in fat was present as unchanged alpha-cypermethrin (Hutson, 1982; Logan, 1983; Hutson & Logan, 1986).

6.1.2 Domestic animals

In a study by Francis & Gill (1991), a formulation containing a mixture of flufenoxuron and alpha-cypermethrin was applied to groups of three sheep. The formulation was applied once, either as a dip diluted at 1:1000 to give a solution of 80 mg flufenoxuron per litre and 60 mg alpha-cypermethrin/litre or as a pour-on solution applied directly to the backs of the sheep giving a dose of 0.15 g active ingredient flufenoxuron and 0.2 g alpha-cypermethrin per sheep. The sheep were killed at 3, 7 and 14 days after application and samples of subcutaneous fat, fleece and sheep skin were analysed. The residues of alpha-cypermethrin in fat ranged from < 0.01 to 0.04 mg/kg and in skin from 0.02 to 1.4 mg/kg over the three sampling periods, and they were lower for pour-on formulations than for the dip. Highest tissue residues were found in wool (sampled from the back); these were (for the 3, 7 and 14 day sampling periods, respectively) 730, 1020 and 360 mg/kg for dip application and 360, 440 and 360 mg/kg for pour-on application. Wool sampled from the side of sheep treated with pour-on formulation were 10 to 30 times lower than wool sampled from the back region; with the dip solution, however, wool from the side region contained higher residues than that from the back. Pour-on application gave lower residues than after a dip.

A trial was carried out during 1987 in the United Kingdom in which Friesian/Hereford calves (in total 17 female animals) were treated with an alpha-cypermethrin pour-on formulation. Ten ml of a 16 g/litre formulation was applied to calves along the mid-dorsal line from shoulder to tail. At 3, 7 and 14 days following treatment, animals were sacrificed for analysis of tissues, i.e. perirenal and subcutaneous fat, muscle, kidneys and liver. No residues were detected in muscle and liver samples at any time (limit of determination, 0.01 mg/kg). In the kidneys a maximum of 0.03 mg/kg was found on day 7 but by day 14 the residues had decreased to 0.01 mg/kg or less. The fat tissues contained maximum levels on day 7, i.e. mean concentrations of 0.26 mg/kg (perirenal fat) and 0.08 mg/kg (subcutaneous fat). By day 14 these concentrations had decreased by about two and a half times (Sherren, 1988a) (see also section 5.2.3).

6.1.3 Humans

Six volunteers (two per dose level) received a single oral dose of 0.25, 0.5 or 0.75 mg alpha-cypermethrin and, after a period of 2-3 weeks, five successive daily doses of 0.25, 0.5 or 0.75 mg to study the urinary excretion and bioaccumulation of alpha-cypermethrin. A parallel study with cypermethrin itself was carried out for comparison purposes. The metabolism and rate of excretion of a single oral dose of alpha cypermethrin were similar to those of cypermethrin itself. The rate of excretion was dose-related, approximately 43% of the dose of alpha-cypermethrin being excreted in the urine as free or conjugated *cis*-cyclopropane carboxylic acid (*cis*-CPA) during the first 24 h. Urinary excretion did not increase with repeated oral dosing; an average of 49% of alpha-cypermethrin was excreted in the urine as free or conjugated *cis*-CPA within 24 h (van Sittert et al., 1985; Eadsforth et al., 1988).

6.2 Metabolic transformation

In a study on Wistar rats using alpha-cypermethrin, ^{14}C-labelled in the benzyl moiety, (see section 6.1.1) no evidence was found for any racemization of the chiral centres of alpha-cypermethrin in the residues in intestines, faeces or fat. The major urinary metabolite was the sulfate conjugate of 3-(4-hydroxyphenoxy)benzoic acid, and smaller amounts of 3-phenoxybenzoic acid (II) and 3-(4-hydroxyphenoxy)benzoic acid (III) were identified. In the faeces, 75% of the radioactivity in the extract was unchanged alpha-cypermethrin; minor metabolites included a dihydroxy metabolite (V), 3-(4-hydroxyphenoxy)benzoic acid (III), 3-phenoxybenzoic acid (II) and the 4-hydroxyphenoxy metabolite (IV). In the adipose tissue, the ^{14}C label was mainly associated with unchanged alpha-cypermethrin, but a lipophilic metabolite of either alpha-cypermethrin or 3-phenoxybenzoic acid, probably a mixture of 3-phenoxybenzoyl diacylglycerols, was also present (Hutson, 1982; Logan, 1983; Hutson & Logan, 1986) (see Fig. 2).

6.3 *In vitro* metabolic transformation

Creedy & Logan (1984) studied the *in vitro* metabolism of cypermethrin and alpha-cypermethrin using liver microsomal preparations from rats, rabbits and humans. In order to obtain information on the relative importance of the oxidative and esteric pathways of degradation of these compounds, incubations were carried out both in the presence and absence of an NADPH-generating system. Both cypermethrin and alpha-cypermethrin were broken down via esteric and oxidative pathways by the liver preparations from the three species. For rabbit and human liver microsomes, oxidation was a minor metabolic route compared to esteric hydrolysis in the case of both compounds. Human liver

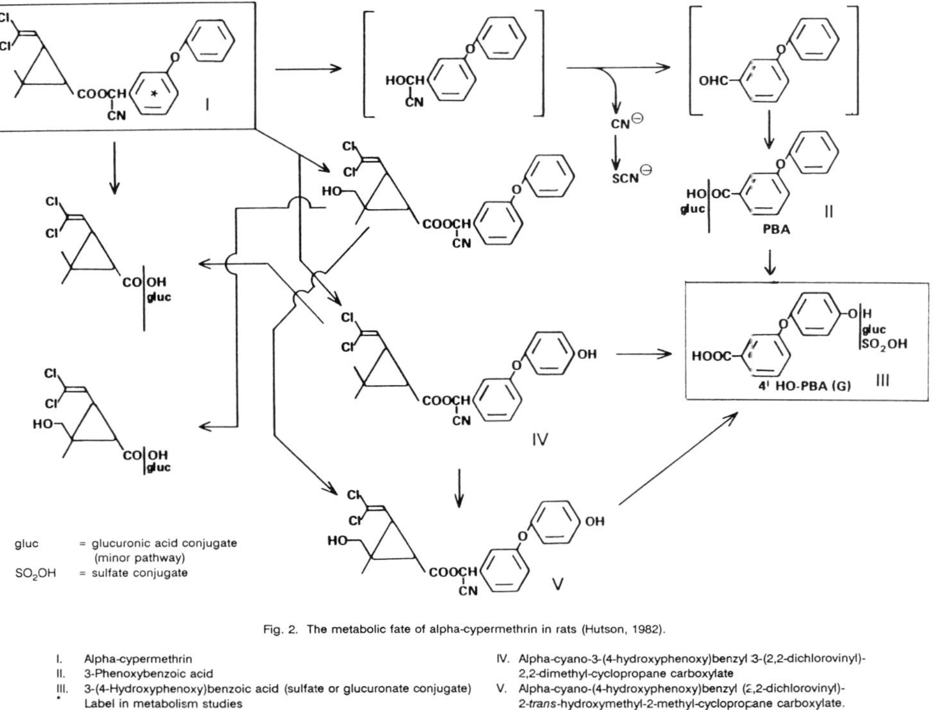

Fig. 2. The metabolic fate of alpha-cypermethrin in rats (Hutson, 1982).

I. Alpha-cypermethrin
II. 3-Phenoxybenzoic acid
III. 3-(4-Hydroxyphenoxy)benzoic acid (sulfate or glucuronate conjugate)
* Label in metabolism studies
IV. Alpha-cyano-3-(4-hydroxyphenoxy)benzyl 3-(2,2-dichlorovinyl)-2,2-dimethyl-cyclopropane carboxylate
V. Alpha-cyano-(4-hydroxyphenoxy)benzyl (2,2-dichlorovinyl)-2-*trans*-hydroxymethyl-2-methyl-cyclopropane carboxylate.

microsomes were able to carry out the esteric hydrolysis of alpha-cypermethrin slightly faster than cypermethrin. In the liver preparations of all three species, cyclopropane carboxylic acid (mainly produced via the esteric pathway) was the main metabolite for both compounds (to the extent of approximately 90-99%). Via the oxidative route, mono-hydroxycypermethrins, dihydroxy-cypermethrin and small amounts of hydroxycyclopropane carboxylic acid (rat only) were also produced.

6.4 Plants

The metabolism of cypermethrin in plants is described in WHO (1989).

The degradation of alpha-cypermethrin and cypermethrin in cabbages grown to maturity outdoors has been studied. Eighteen days after transplanting, the cabbages were treated three times with ^{14}C-labelled alpha-cypermethrin or cypermethrin as an EC formulation. Each treatment consisted of 1.8 mg equivalent with a spray concentration of 36 g/litre. This treatment was repeated after 11 and 27 days. Each box of cabbages received a total application of 5.4 mg at a dose rate equivalent to 50 g active ingredient/ha. At harvest (3 months later) the plants were separated into old and new outer leaves, heart, stalk and roots. No major differences between the two compounds in distribution of radioactivity throughout the plants or in the metabolic profile were observed. The highest radioactive residues were present in the old outer leaves (23% for alpha-cypermethrin and 27% for cypermethrin), lower levels being found in new outer leaves, stalk, roots and heart. Very low levels (< 0.05 mg/kg) of both compounds were found in the soil. The major radioactive residue at harvest was shown to be the pesticide, which was either in the unchanged form or had undergone cis/trans-isomerization, presumably photochemically. The profiles of the organosoluble metabolites were similar, and the major products of alpha-cypermethrin had chromatographic mobility similar to previously identified products of cypermethrin metabolism, such as 3-phenoxybenzoic acid and 3-phenoxybenzyl alcohol, partly hydroxylated and/or conjugated. These compounds were found in minor quantities (McMinn, 1983a; WHO, 1989).

Appraisal

A wide range of studies in mice, rats, dogs, sheep, cows and humans has shown that cypermethrin is rapidly absorbed, distributed to a variety of organs and tissues, metabolized and rapidly excreted from the body (WHO, 1989). There are no major differences in the absorption, distribution, retention or excretion between the species. Differences, where they do occur, are related to the rate rather than the nature of the metabolites formed and the conjugation reactions.

Cypermethrin, both the cis and trans isomers, and alpha-cypermethrin are primarily metabolized by cleavage of the ester bond. The metabolites PBA and CPA are mainly excreted as conjugates. The type of conjugate differs in a number of animal species dosed with cypermethrin, but humans and rats have the same pathway. Minor quantities of hydroxylated PBA (conjugated) may also be found. The terminal half-life of elimination of alpha-cypermethrin from the fat of rats is 17-26 days, compared to 18.9 days for cis-cypermethrin.

7. EFFECTS ON LABORATORY MAMMALS AND *IN VITRO* TEST SYSTEMS

7.1 Single exposure

7.1.1 Oral (technical product)

Alpha-cypermethrin is moderately to highly toxic and 3-4 times more toxic than cypermethrin.

The clinical signs of toxicity observed in the various acute toxicity studies on experimental animals with alpha-cypermethrin are typical for a cyano-containing pyrethroid intoxication. They included ataxia, abasia, gait abnormalities, choreoathetosis, "tip-toe" walk, and increased salivation, lacrimation, piloerection, tremor and clonic convulsions. The majority of the mortalities occurred within the first 3 h and surviving animals recovered within 7 days (Rose, 1982, 1983a).

In the study with alpha-cypermethrin administered in corn-oil (Rose, 1983a), clonic convulsions, piloerection, salivation and splayed hind-leg gait were found. The oral LD_{50} values for alpha-cypermethrin are summarized in Table 3.

Table 3. Oral LD_{50} values for technical alpha-cypermethrin

Species (strain)	Concentration and vehicle	LD_{50} in mg/kg body weight (with 95% confidence limits)	Reference
Mouse (CD)	5% in corn oil	35 (26-48)	Rose (1982)
	40% in DMSO	762 (514-912)	Rose (1982)
	50% aqueous suspension	798 (568-1074)	Rose (1982)
Rat (Wistar)	5% in corn oil	79 (63-98)	Dewar (1981)
	40% in DMSO	approximately 4000	Rose (1982)
	50% aqueous suspension	> 5000	Rose (1982)
Rat (Wistar)	10% in corn oil	40-80	Rose (1983a)
	20% in corn oil	368 (282-487)	Rose (1983a)

Woollen et al. (1991) noted a higher degree of absorption of cypermethrin when it was applied in corn oil. This could be the explanation for the higher toxicity of alpha-cypermethrin administered in corn oil.

7.1.2 Oral (formulations)

Formulations of alpha-cypermethrin have moderate acute oral toxicity (Table 4). The clinical signs observed after oral administration to rats are characteristic of cyano-containing pyrethroid intoxication (see section 7.1.1.). The majority of the mortalities occurred within 3 days of dosing. The degree of acute oral toxicity of formulations containing mixtures with other active ingredients depended on the toxicity of the latter ingredients.

7.1.3 Dermal

Alpha-cypermethrin has low dermal toxicity. No deaths or signs of intoxication were observed in rats (Dewar, 1981; Shell, 1983a) and mice (Rose, 1982; Shell, 1983a) receiving a single 24-h dermal exposure of 500 mg/kg body weight (25% in DMSO) and 100 mg/kg body weight (5% in corn oil), respectively.

The dermal LD_{50} values in rats of formulations of alpha-cypermethrin and of alpha-cypermethrin mixed with another active ingredient are summarized in Table 4. In all cases, the maximum dose that could be applied was tested.

With the pour-on formulations, no clinical signs were observed. Blood around the nose and eyes was the only sign seen in the case of SC formulations. Clinical signs observed after the application of EC or ULV formulations of alpha-cypermethrin included increased lacrimation, chromodacryorrhoea and unkempt appearance, aggressiveness and diarrhoea. The Fastac/BPMC formulation caused the same signs of intoxication and also oedema at the application site. With the Fastac/methomyl formulation, fasciculation, lethargy, salivation, piloerection, hunched back, chromodacryorrhoea and cyanosis were observed. Animals treated with Fastac/Azodrin formulation showed the above-mentioned symptoms, and some additionally showed ataxia, abasia, hypothermia, eye pallor and prostration/coma.

7.1.4 Inhalation

Groups of five male and five female albino Fischer-344 rats were exposed for 4 h to a dust atmosphere containing 30% (m/m)

Table 4. Oral and dermal LD_{50} values for formulated alpha-cypermethrin in rats (Fischer-344)

Formulation[a]	LD_{50} in mg total formulation per kg body weight (with 95% confidence limits) Oral	Dermal	Reference
100 g/litre EC	101 (82-119)	> 1800	Rose (1984d)
100 g/litre EC	136 (98-186)	> 1800	Rose (1984e)
100 g/litre EC	174 (125-327)	> 2000	Price (1985a)
30 g/litre EC	229 (178-292)	> 2000	Rose (1984f)
30 g/litre EC	673 (597-753)	> 2000	Rose (1985)
15 g/litre pour-on	> 2000	> 2000	Price (1988)
10 g/litre pour-on	> 2000	> 2000	Price (1988)
100 g/litre SC	1804 (1507-2168)	> 2000	Price (1985b)
60 g/litre SC	> 5000	> 2000	Gardner (1991)
15 g/litre SC	> 5000	> 2000	Price (1986)
15 g/litre ULV	5838 (5130-6665)	> 2000	Rose (1984c)
Mixtures with other active ingredients			
Fastac/methomyl EC 15/120 g/litre	58-97 (males) 73 (51-89) (females)	> 1900 > 1900	Rose (1984h)
Fastac/BPMC[b] EC 10/400 g/litre	310 (215-462)	> 2000	Price (1987)
Fastac/Azodrin EC 20/400 g/litre	25 (18-34)	> 2000	Gardner (1989)

[a] EC = emulsifiable concentrate; SC = suspension concentrate; ULV = ultra-low volume

[b] BPMC = 2 *sec*-butylphenyl methylcarbamate (fenobucarb)

alpha-cypermethrin on silica powder at an average concentration of 1.3 g/m^3 (equivalent to 0.4 g active ingredient/m^3). The mass media diameter of the dust particles was 4.2 μm (geometric standard deviation 6.4). The animals were observed for 14 days after the exposure but there were no signs of intoxication.

Macroscopic examination of the lungs did not reveal any effects. Thus, the acute LC_{50} was > 1.3 g 30% silica powder dust/m³ or > 0.4 g active ingredient/m³ (Blair, 1984).

7.1.5 Other routes

The acute intraperitoneal LD_{50} for rats of a 10% solution of alpha-cypermethrin in corn oil was 3.39 (3.03-3.83) ml/kg body weight, or 339 mg active ingredient per kg body weight. The surviving animals showed characteristic pyrethroid signs of intoxication, e.g., ataxia, abasia, choreoathetosis, gait abnormalities, "tip-toe" walk and salivation (Rose, 1984a).

7.2 Short-term exposure

7.2.1 Oral

7.2.1.1 Rat

Groups of Wistar rats (10 of each sex at each dose level and 20 of each sex as controls) were fed 0, 25, 100, 200, 400 or 800 mg alpha-cypermethrin/kg diet (equivalent to 0, 1.25, 5, 10, 20 or 40 mg/kg body weight) for 5 weeks. At 400 and 800 mg/kg diet, signs of intoxication, such as abnormal gait and hypersensitivity were observed, and food intake and body weight were decreased in both sexes compared with the control group. Changes in blood chemistry, e.g., decreases in protein and increases in urea levels, were observed in both sexes of rats fed 800 mg/kg diet and in males fed 400 mg/kg. The weights of livers and kidneys of both sexes of rats fed 800 mg/kg diet and livers of male rats fed 400 mg/kg were increased. No histopathological changes were observed except in the case of one severely intoxicated male animal fed 800 mg/kg diet, which showed sparse axonal degeneration in the sciatic nerve. No effects were seen in the animals fed 200 mg/kg diet for five weeks (Pickering, 1982).

In a 13-week study, Wistar rats (30 males and 30 females per test group, and a control group consisting of 60 males and 60 females), which were initially 5 weeks old, were fed 0, 20, 60, 180 or 540 mg alpha-cypermethrin/kg diet (equivalent to 0, 1, 3, 9 or 27 mg/kg body weight). After six weeks of feeding, one third of the animals were killed for interim haematological, clinical chemical and gross post-mortem examination. The remaining animals were killed after 13 weeks. Signs of intoxication, such as abnormal gait with splayed hind limbs, were found in 3 out of 20 males fed 540 mg/kg diet. Several instances of transient skin sores and fur loss were observed particularly in the rats fed 540 mg/kg. There was decreased growth, which correlated with decreased food intake, in both sexes fed 540 mg/kg from the first week onwards. No clear effects on the haematological and clinical chemical parameters were found. Organ weights were comparable with those of the control animals. No histopathological abnormalities were found except sparse axonal degeneration in the sciatic nerve, without clinical signs of toxicity, in two males fed 540 mg/kg. No axonopathy was observed in the three animals with abnormal gait. There were marginal effects (decreased growth during week one and from week 10 onwards) in the males fed 180 mg/kg diet. No effects were found in the 60-mg/kg group (Clark, 1982).

7.2.1.2 Dog

Beagle dogs (one male and one female) were fed alpha-cypermethrin in the diet at the following concentrations: 200 mg/kg diet for 7 days, 400 mg/kg diet for 2 days, and 300 mg/kg diet for 7 days. With 200 mg/kg no signs of intoxication were observed, whereas dosing with 300 mg/kg or more caused weight loss, ataxia, subdued behaviour, head nodding, food regurgitation, inflammation of gums and tongue, body tremors and diminished response to stimuli. Haematological, clinical chemical and gross pathological examination showed no effects (Greenough & Goburdhun, 1984).

In a further study, Beagle dogs (one male and one female) received 300 mg/kg diet for 3 days (male dog) or 4 days (female dog) and 250 mg/kg diet for 7 days. Both animals showed the above-mentioned signs of intoxication, the only difference being that when it was being fed the 250-mg/kg diet the female animal showed these signs more frequently than the male animal. There were no effects on haematology, clinical chemical parameters, urinalysis, faecal occult blood test or gross pathology (Greenough & Goburdhun, 1984).

In a study by Greenough et al. (1984), 36 pure bred Beagle dogs (18 males and 18 females) received a diet containing alpha-cypermethrin at 0, 30, 90 or 270 mg/kg diet for 13 weeks. The group dosed at the highest concentration comprised six males and six females while the other groups consisted of four males and four females. All animals fed 270 mg/kg diet exhibited signs of intoxication, such as whole body tremors, head nodding, "lip-licking", subduedness, ataxia, agitation and a high-stepping gait.

These signs increased in both intensity and duration as the study progressed. Food consumption, body weight gain, organ weights, ophthalmoscopy, haematological and clinical chemical parameters, urinalysis, gross pathology and microscopy of 18 organs and tissues of all test groups showed no dose-related effects. In this study, the no-observed-effect level was considered to be 90 mg/kg diet (equivalent to 2.25 mg/kg body weight).

7.3 Skin and eye irritation; sensitization

7.3.1 Skin irritation

Undiluted technical alpha-cypermethrin was minimally irritating when applied as a single occluded dose for 24 h to intact and abraded rabbit skin (Dewar, 1981).

New Zealand white rabbits were used to study the primary skin irritation of a number of alpha-cypermethrin formulations. The test duration was 4 h, the observation period was 7-21 days, and the formulations tested were 30 and 100 g/litre EC, 15 g/litre ULV, 10 and 15 g/litre pour-on formulation, 15 and 100 g/litre SC, and Fastac/methomyl (15/120) EC. The EC formulations caused mild to moderate skin irritation. Superficial necrosis was observed in one or two animals treated with 100 g/litre EC, but there was no permanent in-depth skin damage. The effects persisted for up to 7 days. The EC formulations and the 100 g/litre SC formulation were classified as mildly irritating. All other formulations tested were either non-irritating or only slightly irritating (Rose, 1984c,d,e,f,h, 1985; Price, 1985a,b, 1986, 1988).

7.3.2 Eye irritation

Undiluted formulations were tested for their eye irritancy potential in groups of six rabbits using the Draize test. All the EC formulations tested (30 or 100 g/litre) caused severe eye irritation, including corneal opacity and damage to the iris (Rose, 1984d,e,f, 1985).

When an EC formulation (100 g/litre) and its components, both in the undiluted form and at typical in-use dilutions (1 in 400 and 1 in 1333 aqueous dilution), were tested for eye irritancy potential, the undiluted formulation was severely irritating, with or without irrigation, while the undiluted blank formulations were mildly to severely irritating. The diluted test formulations, with or without alpha-cypermethrin or with emulsifier, were non-irritating. It was concluded that the eye irritation resulted from the combined formulation ingredients (especially the emulsifier) and that alpha-cypermethrin *per se* gave only slight irritation, if any (Dewar, 1981; Rose, 1984b). In-use dilutions (0.0075%) of another 100 g/litre EC formulation and its blank formulation were non-irritating (Rose, 1984g).

Two pour-on formulations (10 and 15 g/litre) caused moderate and slight conjunctival inflammation, respectively. The 10 g/litre formulation was considered to be an eye irritant (Price, 1988). Two SC formulations (15 and 100 g/litre) were mildly irritating, causing slight conjunctival redness and chemosis (Price, 1985b, 1986). A 15 g/litre ULV formulation was mildly irritating to rabbit eyes and there was a moderate initial pain response (Rose, 1984c). An EC formulation containing Fastac/methomyl (15:120 g/litre) was a severe eye irritant. The vascularization of the cornea and iritis were considered to be irreversible (Rose, 1984h).

7.3.3 Sensitization

Technical alpha-cypermethrin was tested in the guinea-pig maximization test of Magnusson and Kligman using groups of 10 male and 10 female guinea-pigs and a control group of 55 animals of each sex. The following concentrations were used: intradermal injection, 0.05% (v/v) in corn oil; topical application and challenge, 50% (m/m) in vaseline. On the basis of the negative results it was concluded that alpha-cypermethrin is not a skin sensitizer in guinea-pigs (Dewar, 1981).

An EC formulation (100 g/litre) and its corresponding blank were tested, as a 50% solution in corn oil, in the Buehler guinea-pig sensitization test. The topical challenge was carried out with a 30% solution in corn oil. None of the animals showed positive responses at 24 or 48 h after the challenge (Rose, 1984g).

7.4 Long-term and carcinogenicity studies

No long-term or carcinogenicity studies have been conducted with alpha-cypermethrin.

7.5 Reproduction, embryotoxicity and teratogenicity

Alpha-cypermethrin has not been tested for reproductive effects or teratogenicity.

From the available reproduction and teratogenicity studies with cypermethrin it is clear that no influence on reproduction performance occurs at a level of 100 mg/kg diet, nor are there any teratogenic effects even with dose levels high enough to cause maternal toxicity (WHO, 1989). Furthermore, the no-observed-effect level of cypermethrin for reproduction and teratogenicity is comparable with the no-observed-effect levels based on other parameters of toxicity. In consequence, there is no reason to believe that alpha-cypermethrin, consisting of two cis isomers also present in cypermethrin, would behave differently.

7.6 Mutagenicity and related end points

7.6.1 *Mutation*

The results of the various mutagenicity studies with alpha-cypermethrin are summarized in Table 5.

Alpha-cypermethrin (in DMSO) at concentrations of 31.25, 62.5, 125, 250, 500, 1000, 2000 or 4000 μg/ml did not increase reverse gene mutation (at the arg 4-17, trp 5-48 or hom 3-10 markers) in log- or stationary-phase cultures or forward mutation (to cyclo-heximide-resistance) in log-phase cultures of *Saccharomyces cerevisiae* XV 185-14C, either in the presence or absence of rat-liver S9 fraction. Concentrations of 10 and 50 μg/ml 4-nitroquinoline-*N*-oxide and 1250 and 5000 μg/ml cyclophosphamide were used as positive controls (Brooks, 1984).

Alpha-cypermethrin (in DMSO) at concentrations of 31.25, 62.5, 125, 250, 500, 1000, 2000 or 4000 μg/plate, both with and without microsomal activation, did not increase reverse mutation rates in *Salmonella typhimurium* TA98, TA100, TA1535, TA1537 and TA1538 or in *Escherichia coli* WP2 and WP2 uvr A. Mitotic gene conversion was not induced in liquid suspension cultures of log-phase cells of *Saccharomyces cerevisiae* JD 1, dosed with solutions of alpha-cypermethrin at concentrations of 10, 100, 500, 1000 or 5000 μg/ml, both in the presence or absence of a rat liver S9 fraction. These studies were carried out in comparison with four positive control compounds (Brooks, 1982).

7.6.2 *Chromosomal effects*

In a study by Clare & Wiggins (1984), groups of five male and five female Wistar rats were administered a single oral dose of 2, 4 or 8 mg alpha-cypermethrin in 5% corn oil/kg body weight and

Table 5. Mutagenicity tests on microorganisms

Organism/strain	Dose	Type of test	Metabolic activation	Result	Reference
Salmonella typhimurium TA98, TA100, TA1535, TA1537, TA1538	up to 4000 μg/plate	plate	with or without	negative	Brooks (1982)
Escherichia coli WP2, WP2 uvrA	up to 4000 μg/plate	plate	with or without	negative	Brooks (1982)
Saccharomyces cerevisiae JDI	up to 5000 μg/ml	liquid suspension culture	with or without	negative	Brooks (1982)
Saccharomyces cerevisiae XV 185-14C	up to 4000 μg/ml	liquid suspension culture	with or without	negative	Brooks (1984)
Rat liver cells (RL4) (chromatid gaps, breaks or aberrations)	up to 40 μg/ml			negative	Brooks (1982)
Rat liver DNA (DNA single strand damage)	one oral dose of 40 mg/kg body weight			negative	Wooder (1982)
Rat bone marrow chromosome study	one oral dose of up to 8 mg/kg body weight			negative	Clare & Wiggins (1984)

killed 24 h after dosing. The control group received corn oil alone. Cyclophosphamide was used as a positive control. Alpha-cypermethrin caused no increase in the incidence of chromatid or chromosome aberrations or polyploidy in bone marrow cells.

Alpha-cypermethrin in aqueous carboxymethylcellulose at concentrations of up to 40 μg/ml did not increase the frequency of chromatid gaps, chromatid breaks or total chromatid aberrations in rat liver (RL4) cell cultures (Brooks, 1982).

7.6.3 DNA damage

Alpha-cypermethrin in DMSO (20%) was administered to Wistar rats as a single oral dose of 40 mg/kg body weight. The exposure time was 6 h. Alpha-cypermethrin failed to produce any detectable DNA single-strand damage using alkaline elution profiles of liver DNA. Methylmethane sulfonate was used as a positive control and DMSO as the solvent control (Wooder, 1982).

7.6.4 Conclusion

From the available data on alpha-cypermethrin, it can be concluded that this compound is non-mutagenic in tests with *Salmonella typhimurium*, *Saccharomyces cerevisiae*, and *in vivo* and *in vitro* tests with rat liver cells for the induction of chromosome aberration and production of DNA single-strand damage.

7.7 Special studies

7.7.1 Skin sensation

It is known that exposure to certain types of pyrethroids can result in a transient skin sensation in humans (Le Quesne et al., 1980).

Guinea-pigs received 0.1 ml of a 0.01, 0.1 or 1.0% solution of alpha-cypermethrin in ethanol or a 1, 10 or 20% solution of alpha-cypermethrin (w/v) in corn oil on the skin. Sensory stimulation was quantified by counting the number of times each animal turned to lick or bite its treated flank in preference to the non-treated flank. Skin stimulation was observed during a 2-h period at all dose levels except the lowest. In the groups of guinea-pigs treated with 10% and 20%, some animals exhibited an exaggerated hopping movement and a repeated head shaking activity at the time of maximum skin stimulation (40-60 min after treatment).

This behaviour was not seen with the 1% solution or more dilute ones (Hend, 1983).

7.7.2 Neurotoxicity

Large oral doses of alpha-cypermethrin and other synthetic pyrethroids (WHO, 1989) have been shown to produce minor histopathological lesions in the sciatic nerve of rats, described as sparse axonopathy in peripheral nerves.

Rose (1983b) conducted a two-phase study. In the first phase, the time-course for development and recovery from pyrethroid-induced nerve lesions was investigated by measuring biochemical correlates of neuropathological change (the enzymes beta-glucuronidase and beta-galactosidase) in groups of Wistar rats (five of each sex per group) at periods of 2-12 weeks after the start of dosing. The daily doses of alpha-cypermethrin (96.6%), administered by stomach tube, were 37.5 mg/kg body weight for the first 11 doses and 25.0 mg/kg body weight for the subsequent 9 doses over a 4-week period (5 times/week). DMSO was used as the solvent for 10 doses and then arachis oil. In all, 21% of the animals died and more than 80% of the treated animals showed clinical signs of intoxication. Maximum enzyme activities in the sciatic posterior tibial nerves were found 5 weeks after the start of the experiment and had returned to control values by 12 weeks. In the trigeminal nerve and trigeminal ganglia, a slight but not significant increase in enzyme activities was found.

In the second phase of the study, 10 male and 10 female Wistar rats were given 20 oral doses of alpha-cypermethrin in DMSO (0, 10, 20 or 40 mg/kg body weight per day) over a period of 4 weeks (5 times/week). Only two animals died, one given 10 mg/kg and one given 20 mg/kg. In the 40-mg/kg group, 75% of the animals developed clinical signs, whereas in the 20-mg/kg group only 25% of the animals showed these clinical effects. In the 10-mg/kg group, the animals showed no differences from the controls. No clear influence of alpha-cypermethrin on growth was found. Five weeks after the initial dose, which corresponded to the period of maximal enzyme changes, biochemical changes (increases of up to 60%) indicative of a mild axonal degeneration were found in both the distal and proximal sections of the sciatic posterior tibial nerve in animals administered 40 mg/kg body weight. In the 20-mg/kg group, only a small (up to 20%) increase in beta-galactosidase activity was found in the proximal sections of the sciatic posterior nerve. The same trends were found in the trigeminal nerve and ganglia. No changes were found in the 10-mg/kg group (Rose, 1983b).

7.7.3 *Immunosuppressive action*

No data on the immunosuppressive action of alpha-cypermethrin are available.

7.8 Mechanism of toxicity - mode of action

The mechanism of toxicity and mode of action of cypermethrin (and other pyrethroids) are extensively described in section 8.8 of the Environmental Health Criteria 82: Cypermethrin (WHO, 1989). Recently Vijverberg & van den Bercken (1990) and Aldridge (1990) summarized current knowledge of the neurotoxicity and mode of action of the different pyrethroids (see also Appendix 1).

Pyrethroids induce toxic signs that are characteristic of a strong excitatory action on the nervous system. Toxic doses generally cause hypersensitivity to sensory stimuli, and a number of compounds may induce tingling sensations in the skin. Two distinct toxic syndromes have been described in mammals. The T-syndrome is induced by pyrethrins and non-cyano pyrethroids, and the CS-syndrome, induced by cyano-pyrethroids such as cypermethrin and alpha-cypermethrin, is characterized by choreoathetosis and salivation.

The available data strongly suggest that the primary target site of pyrethroid insecticides in the vertebrate nervous system is the sodium channel in the nerve membrane. Pyrethroids without an alpha-cyano group cause a moderate prolongation of the transient increase in sodium permeability of the nerve membrane during excitation. This results in relatively short trains of repetitive nerve impulses in sense organs, sensory (afferent) nerve fibres and, in effect, nerve terminals. On the other hand, the alpha-cyano pyrethroids (for instance cypermethrin and alpha-cypermethrin) cause a long-lasting prolongation of the transient increase in sodium permeability of the nerve membrane during excitation. This results in long-lasting trains of repetitive impulses in sense organs and a frequency-dependent depression of the nerve impulse in nerve fibres. The difference in effects between permethrin (with no alpha-cyano group) and the two insecticides cypermethrin and alpha-cypermethrin, which have identical molecular structures except for the presence of an alpha-cyano group on the phenoxybenzyl alcohol, indicates that it is this alpha-cyano group that is responsible for the long-lasting prolongation of the sodium permeability.

Since the mechanisms responsible for nerve impulse generation and conduction are basically the same throughout the entire nervous system, pyrethroids may also induce repetitive activity in various parts of the brain. The difference between the symptoms of poisoning by alpha-cyano pyrethroids and those of the classical pyrethroids is not necessarily due to an exclusive central site of action. It may be related to the long-lasting repetitive activity in sense organs and possibly in other parts of the nervous system, which, in a more advance state of poisoning, may be accompanied by a frequency-dependent depression of the nervous impulse.

Pyrethroids also cause pronounced repetitive activity and a prolongation of the transient increase in sodium permeability of the nerve membrane in insects and other invertebrates. Available information indicates that the sodium channel in the nerve membrane is also the most important target site of pyrethroids in the invertebrate nervous system.

Because of the universal character of the processes underlying nerve excitability, the action of pyrethroids should not be considered to be restricted to particular animal species or to a certain region of the nervous system.

Although it has been established that sense organs and nerve endings are most vulnerable to the action of pyrethroids, the ultimate lesion that causes death will depend on the animal species, environmental conditions, and on the chemical structure and physical characteristics of the pyrethroid molecule.

8. EFFECTS ON HUMANS

8.1 General population exposure

No data concerning the exposure of the general population to alpha-cypermethrin are available.

8.2 Occupational exposure

A study of alpha-cypermethrin exposures was carried out during formulation using both technical concentrate and technical material at Durban, South Africa. The oil-damped solid, crystalline, dry technical concentrate contained a minimum of 90% (m/m) alpha-cypermethrin. Exposures were assessed by personal and static monitoring of atmospheric alpha-cypermethrin concentrations, urinary alpha-cypermethrin metabolite concentrations and by medical examination. Four individuals were exposed during 3 days of operation. The group mean personal exposures for the two days whilst formulating technical concentrate were 2.8 and 4.9 $\mu g/m^3$ and the group mean personal exposure to technical material on day 3 was 54.1 $\mu g/m^3$. Urinary alpha-cypermethrin metabolites could not be identified (limit of detection, 0.02 mg/litre). Formulation was successfully completed, only minor skin sensations being reported by two of the non-operational personnel, possibly resulting from particles of alpha-cypermethrin settling directly on the skin, face and neck. Dust concentrations were up to 30 times greater during handling the technical material compared with oil-damped technical concentrate, and local exhaust dust extraction reduced dust emission by a factor of up to 17 (Western, 1984).

9. EFFECTS ON OTHER ORGANISMS IN THE LABORATORY AND FIELD

Appraisal

The acute toxicity of alpha-cypermethrin to Daphnia magna *and* Gammarus pulex *is similar to that of cypermethrin. However, in a reproduction study with* Daphnia magna, *alpha-cypermethrin seemed to be slightly more toxic than cypermethrin. Comparison of the results of a reproduction study in* Daphnia magna *with the results of acute tests shows that the hazard of alpha-cypermethrin lies in its acute toxicity. There is no significant potential for cumulative effects occurring as a result of long-term exposure to lower concentrations.*

Alpha-cypermethrin is highly toxic to a number of aquatic arthropod taxa but of low toxicity to molluscs. The short-term toxicity of the compound can be reduced by formulating the product as an OSC. Contamination through spray drift from commercial applications will generally be low, and so the effects on susceptible taxa will be limited. The rapid loss of alpha-cypermethrin from the water gives the potential for complete recovery of affected populations.

Laboratory studies show that values for the acute toxicity and the toxicity to the early-life stages of fish are similar for alpha-cypermethrin and cypermethrin. A comparison of the results from both alpha-cypermethrin studies reveals that the hazard of the compound results from its acute toxicity, and there is no significant potential for additional effects occurring as a result of long-term exposure to lower concentrations. Laboratory and field studies have shown that the toxicity of alpha-cypermethrin to fish is greatly influenced by the formulation, particulate formulations showing significantly less toxicity than emulsifiable concentrates.

Field studies demonstrate that the high toxicity of alpha-cypermethrin to fish observed in laboratory studies is not realized under field conditions. Contamination of water bodies by inadvertent overspraying or spray drift does not present a hazard to fish.

9.1 Microorganisms

9.1.1 Algae

The acute toxicity of alpha-cypermethrin to a single-celled green alga, *Selenastrum capricornutum*, at 24 °C has been determined. The pesticide was dispersed using acetone, and the 2- to 4-day EC_{50} for growth was above 100 μg/litre (Stephenson, 1982).

9.1.2 Bacteria

The effects of cypermethrin on microbial activity in the soil have been investigated in a series of studies. Cypermethrin was applied to sandy loam at concentrations of 2.5 and 250 mg/kg. No effects on the rates of carbon dioxide evolution or oxygen uptake were observed at the lower rate, but significant inhibition of carbon dioxide evolution and a decrease in oxygen uptake were observed at the higher rate of application. There were no effects at either concentration on nitrogen fixation, ammonification, nitrification or glucose utilization (WHO, 1989).

Sewage bacteria were unaffected by the presence of alpha-cypermethrin (3 mg/litre) in a closed system test, while the growth of *Pseudomonas fluorescens* was unaffected at 100 mg/litre (Stone & Watkinson, 1983).

9.2 Aquatic organisms

9.2.1 Invertebrates

9.2.1.1 Laboratory studies

Acute toxicity studies with *Daphnia magna* (aged < 24 h) showed that at 20 °C technical alpha-cypermethrin, dispersed in acetone under static conditions (daily renewal), has effects at concentrations below 1 μg/litre. The 24-h and 48-h EC_{50} values (immobilization) were 1.1 and 0.3 μg/litre, respectively (Stephenson, 1982).

Water samples taken from field enclosures 24 h after treatment with an EC formulation were analysed for alpha-cypermethrin and bioassayed with *Gammarus pulex*. The 24-h LC_{50} value for this organism was 0.05 μg/litre (Garforth, 1982a; Shires, 1982).

The effect of technical alpha-cypermethrin on survival, growth and reproduction of *Daphnia magna* was studied over a period of 21 days by Garforth (1982b). The test solution was renewed daily and the temperature ranged between 18.5 and 20.2 °C. The results are summarized in Table 6.

Table 6. Effects of alpha-cypermethrin on the reproductive cycle of *Daphnia magna*[a]

Effect	Nominal concentration (µg/litre) LOEL	NOEL
Survival of parent generation	0.3	0.1
Growth of parent generation	0.1	0.03
Production of young	0.1	0.03

[a] From: Garforth (1982b)
LOEL = Lowest-observed-effect level; NOEL = No-observed-effect level

9.2.1.2 Field studies

Garforth (1982a) studied the effects of alpha-cypermethrin on a range of aquatic invertebrates in metal enclosures, each containing about 1 m^3 water, placed in an outdoor experimental pond. A diluted EC formulation was sprayed onto the water surface at concentrations of 1, 3, 10, 30 and 100 g active ingredient/ha, and samples were taken up to 7 days after application. The concentration of alpha-cypermethrin was around 50% of the nominal level 24 h after application and decreased to 10 to 20% of the nominal level 7 days after application. The lowest concentration was toxic to *Asellidae*. Thirteen families of aquatic arthropods were tested; most were killed at 1 g/ha except one species of *Coenagriidae*, which tolerated about 3 g/ha. Three families of molluscs were tested and were found to be unaffected at 100 g/ha.

Studies to investigate the relative toxicity of two formulations of alpha-cypermethrin (a 100-g/litre EC and a 100-g/litre oil-enhanced suspension concentrate (OSC) with and without anti-evaporant agents) to aquatic invertebrates have been carried out. Water samples were taken from field enclosures treated with a range of doses (0.1-5 g/ha for the EC and 0.1-10 g/ha for the two OSC formulations) and bioassayed with *Gammarus pulex*. The 24-h LD_{50} values (in g alpha-cypermethrin/ha equivalents) of water samples taken 24 h after application were 0.9 for the EC, 6.3 for the OSC without anti-evaporant, and 2.8 for the OSC plus anti-evaporant formulation. Thus, one day after treatment, both

OSC formulations were less toxic to *Gammarus pulex* than the EC formulation. However, the EC formulation lost its toxicity more rapidly than either of the OSC formulations (see also section 4.1.2). The effects on other aquatic invertebrate communities could not be accurately assessed, since the results for macro-arthropods and zooplankton were inconclusive. *Coenagriidae, Chironomidae* and zooplankton seemed to be relatively tolerant. The residues in water and sediment, 22 days after treatment with the EC at 2 g alpha-cypermethrin/ha or with both OSC formulations at 5 g/ha, were < 0.004 µg/litre and < 0.01 mg/kg, respectively, for all three formulations (Inglesfield, 1985b).

The hazard to aquatic invertebrates resulting from spray drift from the aerial application of an EC (15 g alpha-cypermethrin/ha) has been investigated by Garforth & Woodbridge (1984). Details of the study are described in section 9.2.2.2. The sub-surface water concentration was 0.6 µg alpha-cypermethrin/litre shortly after application and decreased to < 0.02 µg/litre within 2 to 4 days. The contamination initially caused a significant reduction in the abundance of several groups of aquatic arthropods, including beetles, chironomids, corixids, mites and zooplankton. However, within 4 to 7 weeks the affected fauna had completely recovered.

In a study by Pearson (1990), two freshwater ponds were treated with alpha-cypermethrin as an emulsifiable concentrate in 1987. One pond was oversprayed at 15 g active ingredient/ha, while the other was treated with the same amount of alpha-cypermethrin but by direct incorporation into the water (see section 4.1.2). Indigenous populations of zooplankton nauplii and of copepods (*Cyclops* spp.) were significantly reduced in both ponds by the treatment but recovered within 26-45 days. Other zooplankton were not plentiful but appeared to be less severely affected in the oversprayed pond than in the pond treated by incorporation. Populations of phantom midge larvae (*Chaoborus* spp) were killed by both treatments. However, within 47 days after treatment, populations of young larvae had developed in the oversprayed pond to almost pre-treatment numbers, and to a lesser extent in the pond with direct incorporation.

9.2.2 Fish

9.2.2.1 Laboratory studies

The available acute 96-h LC_{50} values for two fish species are summarized in Table 7.

Table 7. Acute toxicity of technical alpha-cypermethrin in fish

Species	Mean weight (g)	Vehicle	Test system	Temperature (°C)	96-h LC_{50} (µg/litre) (95% confidence limits)	Reference
Rainbow trout (*Oncorhynchus mykiss*)	3.3	dispersed via acetone	static water; 12 h renewal of test solutions	15	2.8 (2.1-3.5)	Stephenson (1982)
Fathead minnow (*Pimephales promelas*)	0.76	adsorbed onto pumice	continuous flow-through	23-25	0.93 (0.78-1.2)	Stephenson (1983)

The effects of the type of formulation on the acute toxicity to fish are summarized in Table 8. Suspension concentrate, wettable powder and micro-encapsulated formulations were 10 to 70 times less acutely toxic to rainbow trout than the EC formulation (Shires, 1983b).

Table 8. Effect of type of formulation on the toxicity of alpha-cypermethrin to fish in laboratory studies

Species	Weight (g)	Tempera-ture (°C)	Formulation	96-h LC_{50} (µg/litre)	Reference
Rainbow trout (*Oncorhynchus mykiss*)	0.8-2.5	15	100 g/litre EC	5.6	Shires (1983b)
			250 g/litre SC	350	
			100 g/kg WP	120	
			50 g/kg WP	220	
			50 g/kg ME	> 100	
			50 g/kg CD	65	
Rainbow trout (*Oncorhynchus mykiss*)	0.11-0.25	15	15 g/litre OSC	10[a]	Pearson (1986)
			15 g/litre OSC	71	
			100 g/litre OSC	16[a]	
			100 g/litre OSC	56	
Common carp (*Cyprinus carpio*)	3.5-4	24-30	100 g/litre OSC	11	Stephenson (1986)
			15 g/litre EC	0.8	
			50 g/kg WP	60	
Puntius gonionotus	0.3-0.5	24-30	100 g/litre OSC	3.2	Stephenson (1986)
			15 g/litre EC	0.7	
			50 g/kg WP	22	

[a] Denotes daily renewal of test solutions. All other tests were carried out without renewal of the test solutions.
EC = emulsifiable concentrate; SC = suspension concentrate; OSC = oil-enhanced suspension concentrate; WP = wettable powder; ME = micro-encapsulated; CD = β-cyclodextrin.

The toxicity of alpha-cypermethrin to the early-life stages of fish has been studied in a 34-day continuous-flow embryo-larval test with the fathead minnow (*Pimephales promelas*). Eggs less than 24 h old were exposed to nominal concentrations of 0.03 to 1.0 µg/litre. Pre-hatch, post-hatch and overall mortality and final body weight were recorded. On the basis of the most sensitive parameter (overall survival) and measured exposure concentrations, the lowest concentration of alpha-cypermethrin producing an adverse effect was 0.09 μg/litre and the highest concentration producing no effect (NOEL) was 0.03 μg/litre (Stephenson, 1983).

9.2.2.2 *Small scale field or outdoor tank studies*

The acute effect of formulation on the toxicity of alpha-cypermethrin to fish under field conditions was investigated in studies using stainless steel enclosures placed in an experimental pond. In the first study (Shires, 1983b), the rainbow trout (13-32 g) was the test species and the results are summarized in Table 9. The EC formulation was at least 30 times more toxic than any of the other formulations. The number of fish used was not reported.

Table 9. Effect of formulation on the toxicity of alpha-cypermethrin to rainbow trout in field studies

Formulation	14-day LD_{50} (g active ingredient/ha equivalent)
100 g/litre emulsifiable concentrate	29
250 g/litre suspension concentrate	> 1000
100 g/kg wettable powder	> 1000
50 g/kg micro-encapsulated	> 1000

In the second study, Stephenson (1987c) tested an 1.5% oil-enriched SC formulation of alpha-cypermethrin in outdoor tanks containing carp (*Cyprinus carpio*; 6.3 g). The application rate was approximately 4, 8 and 15-16 g active ingredient/ha applied by hand sprayer. The water temperature ranged from 23-26 °C, the water was aerated and the duration of the experiment was 7 days. There was 20% mortality at all treatment rates, which was comparable with the control group. The number of fish used was not reported.

In the third study (Shires, 1985b), rainbow trout (*Oncorhynchus mykiss*; 2-5 g) were introduced into open-ended stainless steel enclosures placed in a mature experimental pond. Different volumes of alpha-cypermethrin (as a diluted EC containing 100 g active ingredient/litre) were applied with a hand-held sprayer onto the water surface. The dose rates were equivalent to 5-500 g active ingredient/ha. The concentrations in the water samples were dependent on the dose applied and the time after the treatment that the samples were taken. For instance, with a dose of 5 g alpha-cypermethrin/ha the concentration in the water was 0.4 μg/litre or less after 96 h, whereas with a dose of 500 g/ha residues of up to 30 μg/litre were found. Alpha-cypermethrin was toxic to the rainbow trout at a concentration of about 2-5 μg/litre water. In terms of nominal application rate, the no-observed-effect level for alpha-cypermethrin lies between 50 and 100 g alpha-cypermethrin/ha. These dose rates are much higher than those used for crop protection purposes.

In a further study, 20 rainbow trout were placed in stainless steel enclosures in a shallow pond. The diluted EC and SC formulations were sprayed onto the surface of the water and the fish were monitored for mortality over 8 days. The SC formulation did not cause mortality, even at an application rate equivalent to 300 g active ingredient/ha. However, high mortality (90%) occurred with the EC formulation at 30 g/ha alpha-cypermethrin, but application of 10 g active ingredient/ha did not cause mortality. From these results it is clear that the SC formulation has a lower toxicity than the EC formulation (Stephenson, 1987b).

The hazard to fish caused by spray drift from aerial applications of alpha-cypermethrin to agricultural land has been investigated by Garforth & Woodbridge (1984). The trial site was a cereal field bordered on one side by a freshwater ditch. The water's edge was generally less than 2 m from the crop margin. Four days prior to application, two cages, each containing 15 common carp (*Cyprinus carpio*; 30-50 cm) were placed in the ditch. The ditch was known to contain a good stock of different types of fish, macroinvertebrates and zooplankton. An alpha-cypermethrin EC containing 100 g/litre was applied by air at 15 g active ingredient/ha to the crop when a gentle breeze was blowing from the crop over the ditch. The alpha-cypermethrin concentration in the sub-surface water was 0.6 μg/litre shortly after the application and decreased to < 0.02 μg/litre within 2 to 4 days (see section 4.1.2.). None of the fish died and no adverse effects were observed either on the carp placed in the cages or on the indigenous species. It was concluded that inadvertent contamination of water bodies by spray drift resulting from the normal commercial use of alpha-cypermethrin does not present a hazard to fish.

Several field tests in rice paddies have examined the toxicity of alpha-cypermethrin to fish.

Stephenson (1986, 1987b) investigated the acute toxicity of 15 g/litre EC, 100 g/litre OSC and 50 g/kg WP formulations to fish in plots of rice paddy in West Java. The application rates were 7.5, 15, and 30 g alpha-cypermethrin/ha for the EC and OSC formulations and 30 g alpha-cypermethrin/ha for the WP formulation. Each of the insecticide treatments was applied to the same plot on two separate occasions; once 12 days after transplantation of the rice seedlings and again 57 days after the transplantation. Prior to application, two cages each containing 20 carp (*Cyprinus carpio*) (2.5-5 g) and two cages each containing 20 specimens of *Puntius gonionotus* (1.4-5 g) were placed in trenches cut in each plot. In addition, before the first experiment, 30 fish of each of these two species were released to swim freely in each plot. Survival of the fish was monitored daily up to 7 days after each treatment. The water temperature was between 25 and 36 °C. Following the first application, only the EC formulation at 15 and 30 g/ha resulted in significant mortality of caged and free-swimming carp and *Puntius gonionotus*. The same was true for carp following the second application, but no results were available for *Puntius gonionotus* following the second application due to an outbreak of disease among these fish.

Two other field studies were carried out in West Java to examine the effects of an OSC formulation on the growth and survival of free-swimming carp (6-8 g) in rice paddies. Experimental conditions were similar to those described above for the acute studies. The water temperature was 23-32 °C. In the first experiment, treatments with 15 g active ingredient/ha were carried out 21 and 33 days after transplantation of the rice seedlings. In the second experiment, the same dose rate was applied 51 and 64 days after transplanting. The fish were monitored over periods of 3 to 4 weeks in each experiment. No adverse effects on survival and growth of the carp were observed (Stephenson, 1987a,b).

9.3 Terrestrial organisms

9.3.1 *Earthworms*

The toxicity of technical alpha-cypermethrin to the red earthworm, *Eisenia foetida*, has been assessed in laboratory tests. In the filter paper contact toxicity test, 50% mortality occurred within 48 h at a dose of about 0.01 mg/cm^2 of filter paper. However, increases in the dose up to 1 mg/cm^2 did not result in a significant increase in mortality. In the artificial soil test no significant mortality occurred within a period of 14 days in earthworms exposed to up to 100 mg alpha-cypermethrin/kg soil (Inglesfield & Sherwood, 1983).

9.3.2 Invertebrates - field studies

In a study designed to investigate the effects of alpha-cypermethrin on non-target arthropod fauna in Italian vineyards, two formulations of alpha-cypermethrin were tested, i.e. an emulsifiable concentrate (100 g active ingredient/litre) and a suspension concentrate (250 g active ingredient/litre). Both were diluted to 1.25 g active ingredient/ha and sprayed to run-off. The effect on predators and parasites (crop foliage fauna) such as parasitoid *Hymenoptera*, *Heteroptera* and *Chrysopa carnea*, soil surface predators such as *Coleoptera* and *Araneae*, phytophagous arthropods such as *Homoptera*, *Thysanoptera* and *Acari*, and other invertebrates such as nematocerous, Diptera and epigeal fauna was inconclusive but in most cases negative. Spiders were the only group significantly affected by alpha-cypermethrin. The abundance of major phytophagous insect taxa (*Homoptera*, *Thysanoptera* and *Acari*) was markedly reduced by both treatments although neither treatment had any long-term adverse effects (Inglesfield, 1984).

An emulsifiable concentrate (EC) of alpha-cypermethrin was tested on the non-target arthropod fauna of maize in France at 20 and 30 g active ingredient/ha and applied using tractor-mounted boom and nozzle equipment at different stages of crop development. Organisms from the following taxa were collected: phytophagous arthropods (*Aphidoidea*), *Thysanoptera* (*Thripidae*), *Cicadellidae* and entomophagous arthropods; predatory *Coleoptera* (*Coccinellidae*, *Cantharidae*, *Carabidae* and *Staphylinidae*); parasitoid *Hymenoptera* (*Braconidae*, *Chalcidoidea*); and predatory *Diptera*, *Neuroptera* and *Aranea*. In addition, the effects on community structure were studied. The two treatments reduced transiently the numbers of some of the entomophagous taxa, especially *Coccinellidae* (*Coleoptera*), *Carabidae* (*Coleoptera*), *Neuroptera* and *Araneae*. Alpha-cypermethrin at a concentration of 20 g/ha promoted some late-season resurgence of aphid populations (Inglesfield, 1985a).

A large-scale replicated field experiment was carried out in Indonesia to investigate the effects of an EC (10 g and 20 g alpha-cypermethrin/ha) and an OSC (10 g and 20 g alpha-cypermethrin per ha), applied at 17 and 62 days after transplanting using a single fan-jet nozzle knapsack sprayer, on rice pests and their natural enemies. Alpha-cypermethrin was applied at two crop stages, and populations of both pests and beneficial arthropods were monitored throughout the season. Alpha-cypermethrin produced good control of stemborers, grasshoppers, leafhoppers and stinkbugs, the most numerous pests found during the trial. It had a significant but short-lived effect on spiders and, generally, no effect on either dragon-flies or other beneficial arthropods (Shires & Inglesfield, 1986).

A study was initiated in England in 1982 to compare the effects on entomophagous arthropods of annual applications of an EC of alpha-cypermethrin (at a rate of 10 g active ingredient/ha in the first year and 15 g active ingredient/ha in subsequent years) with those resulting from the use of non-pyrethroid products. The study was carried out on a range of crops (oilseed rape, wheat and barley) over the duration of a 5-year arable crop rotation. A field of 8 ha was divided into two equal areas, and each year alpha-cypermethrin was applied to one of the areas and other products to the other area. All treatments were carried out with standard tractor-driven boom and nozzle spraying equipment. The crop rotation was as follows: winter rape in 1982, winter wheat in 1983 and 1984, and winter barley in 1985. Organisms from a variety of taxa were collected during the study, such as parasitoid *Hymenoptera*, predatory *Diptera*, predatory *Coleoptera*, *Araneae*, phytophagous insects and other arthropods. The results indicated that any difference between the effects of alpha-cypermethrin and the reference compounds on entomophagous arthropods was generally short-lived. There is no evidence that alpha-cypermethrin treatments had any long-term effects on any of the taxa studied. In addition, there appeared to be no long-term effects on the relative abundance of entomophages within the arthropod communities or on the structure and integrity of the arthropod communities of which they form a part (Inglesfield, 1985c, 1988, 1989).

The results of these studies have been reviewed by Inglesfield (1991). They showed that field application of alpha-cypermethrin and cypermethrin had no adverse effects on the relative abundance of entomophages within the arthropod communities and that the use of these two pesticides in small grain cereals would not be associated with pest "resurgence" or the development of secondary pest infestations.

9.3.3 Honey-bees

9.3.3.1 Laboratory studies

The oral administration of alpha-cypermethrin in acetone produced a 24-h LD_{50} of 0.06 μg/bee, whereas an EC formulation (100 g/litre) of the pesticide yielded a 24-h LD_{50} of 0.13 μg formulation/bee. After topical application, 24-h LD_{50} values of 0.03 μg (technical) and 0.11 μg (EC) per bee were obtained (Murray, 1985).

The mortality of honey-bees (*Apis mellifera*) exposed to *Phacelia* flowers 30 min after they had been treated with an EC formulation (15 g active ingredient/ha) in a residual test was low (15%) within 48 h. However, the foraging activity was reduced (Murray, 1985).

The residual toxicity to the honey-bee of alpha-cypermethrin as EC, OSC, and EC/fungicide mixtures has been investigated. Bees were exposed for 48 h to flowering *Phacelia campanularia* plants that had been sprayed with each formulation at a rate of 10 or 20 g active ingredient/ha, and the mortality was assessed 24 and 48 h after initial exposure to the treated plants. Although there was great variation in the results, there appeared to be no difference in the residual toxicity of the EC and OSC formulations at a rate of 10 g active ingredient/ha. However, at 20 g active ingredient/ha the OSC appeared to be more toxic than the EC. Application of the EC in admixtures did not appear to significantly increase bee mortality (Hillaby & Inglesfield, 1986).

9.3.3.2 Field studies

Alpha-cypermethrin, applied as an EC (10 and 20 g active ingredient/ha) by tractor-mounted boom and nozzle equipment to small plots of flowering mustard in France, caused a sharp decline in foraging activity of bees immediately after application, but there was a return to normal activity within a few hours. No effect on bee survival or hive development was observed (Shires, 1983a; Shires et al., 1984b; Shires, 1985a).

In a further study, the same EC formulation was applied at the same concentration on large isolated fields of flowering oilseed rape during peak foraging activity of honey-bees in France. No increase in bee mortality was found, but foraging activity declined for a few hours after application at a rate of 10 g active ingredient/ha. With a rate of 20 g active ingredient/ha a more prolonged decline in foraging activity occurred. No effects on the overall condition of the hives were seen at the end of the season and very low or undetectable residues were found in dead bees, pollen, honey and wax (Shires et al., 1984c; Shires, 1985a).

Two large and two small plots of winter wheat were enclosed beneath large mesh-covered tunnels. A small bee-hive was placed in each tunnel and sucrose solution was sprayed onto all of the wheat in order to simulate aphid honey dew. Alpha-cypermethrin (an EC at 10, 15 or 30 g active ingredient/ha) was applied to the larger plots of wheat when the bees were actively foraging the sugar deposits. No increase in bee mortality, compared with that in the pre-treatment period, was observed. Foraging activity in the plots declined sharply after treatment and remained at a reduced level, probably because of its repellent effect. Examination of the hives about 2 weeks after the trial showed that the hives, both the control and the alpha-cypermethrin-treated, were in excellent condition with strong adult populations and large areas of developing brood. In post-treatment samples, alpha-cypermethrin residues of 0.03 mg/kg of honey and 0.01 mg/kg of wax were found. In live and dead bees collected from the tunnel treated with 15 g/ha, a concentration of 0.026 μg/bee was found (Shires et al., 1984a; Le Blanc, 1985).

In a study by Inglesfield & Forbes (1986), alpha-cypermethrin was applied as an OSC (10 g active ingredient/ha) and an EC (10 g active ingredient/ha) to three fields of flowering winter-sown oilseed rape in Germany while bees were actively foraging the crops. None of the treatments had any significant effect on adult bee survival or on the longer-term development of the experimental colonies. The number of bees actively foraging in the crops declined following application. This reduction in activity can probably be partly attributed to the repellent effects of these treatments. Both the OSC and EC formulations of alpha-cypermethrin had similar effects on bee behaviour. Residues of alpha-cypermethrin in post-treatment samples of pollen, honey and wax were below 0.01 mg/kg. In dead bees, the residue on the day of application with the OSC was 1.8 mg/kg and in the case of the EC was 0.12 mg/kg.

A diluted EC formulation of alpha-cypermethrin (mixed with the fungicide vinclozolin, 100 g active ingredient/ha) was applied by a tractor-driven boom and nozzle sprayer, at a rate of 20 g active ingredient/ha, to a 206-ha block of flowering oilseed rape situated in Kent, England. Shortly before spraying, which took place over a 3-day period, five beehives were positioned at each of two sites adjacent to the crop. At each site the hives were either fitted with pollen traps or with traps to collect dead bees as they were removed from the hive. The hives were observed daily before and for ten days after spraying. Hive activity was recorded at intervals each day, and, on days when bees were flying, pollen traps were set and samples of pollen collected. Following the application of alpha-cypermethrin the bees foraged normally. At least 90% of the pollen returned to the hives during the immediate post-treatment period was found to be from oilseed rape, showing that the bees had continued to forage on the treated crop. The number of dead bees collected remained low throughout the study and did not increase after application of the alpha-cypermethrin. After the study, all hives were in good condition and subsequently yielded a good crop of honey. A local beekeeper with many hives adjacent to the same block of oilseed rape reported no effects amongst his hives. It was concluded that the application of alpha-cypermethrin at 20 g active ingredient/ha to flowering oilseed rape had no direct effects on honey-bee survival and hive development (Brown, 1989).

9.3.4 Leaf-cutting bees

Laboratory trials using 15 male adult alfalfa leaf-cutting bees (*Megachile rotundata* F.) per group, exposed to treated filter papers for 4 h, showed that alpha-cypermethrin EC (100 g/litre) at the rate of 10 or 15 g active ingredient/ha caused 12 and 30% mortality, respectively, and 42 and 100% mortality after 24 h of contact (Tasei et al., 1987).

In a study by Tasei et al. (1987), populations of about 400 female alfalfa leaf-cutting bees were reared in three flowering lucerne fields. One field was left untreated, while the two others were treated with alpha-cypermethrin as an EC (10 or 15 g active ingredient/ha), applied by a tractor-mounted fan-jet sprayer. Two days after the treatments, counts of live females in artificial nesting sites showed the losses due to 10 and 15 g active ingredient/ha to be 21 and 12%, respectively. After hibernation and incubation of the progeny larvae, little effect of the treatments could be observed. The maximum residue in leaves collected from nests was 1 mg alpha-cypermethrin/kg. The mean values after 5, 10 and 27 days in leaf pieces capping the nests of the bees were 0.75, 0.48, and 0.19 mg/kg at the lower application rate and 0.59, 0.53, and 0.10 mg/kg at the higher rate. No residues (limit of determination, 0.01 mg/kg) were detected in live larvae but 0.07 mg/kg was found in pollen provisions (Tasei et al., 1987).

9.3.5 Birds

Cypermethrin is practically non-toxic to birds; acute oral LD_{50} values are greater than 2000 mg/kg body weight. The dietary LC_{50} value is above 10 000 mg/kg diet (see WHO, 1989). However, studies with alpha-cypermethrin have not been carried out.

10. COMPARISON BETWEEN ALPHA-CYPERMETHRIN AND CYPERMETHRIN

Alpha-cypermethrin comprises one quarter of the racemic mixture cypermethrin, with which an extensive agricultural, ecological and (eco)toxicological programme has been carried out (WHO, 1989). It contains more than 90% of the insecticidally most active enantiomer pair of the four cis isomers of cypermethrin, i.e. the two cis isomers (IR*cis*)S and (IS*cis*)R (see Fig. 1).

10.1 Use and residue levels

Alpha-cypermethrin is used to control the same pests in agriculture as cypermethrin. Its rate of application to crops (5-30 g active ingredient/ha) is lower than that of cypermethrin (10-200 g active ingredient/ha) since alpha-cypermethrin is biologically more active than cypermethrin.

Residue data for alpha-cypermethrin have been obtained from a large number of supervised trials carried out worldwide. These trials cover the most important crop groupings for which alpha-cypermethrin is recommended, including oilseeds, pome fruits, peaches, fruiting vegetables, berries, leafy vegetables, maize and speciality crops such as hops and tobacco (Shell, 1984). Residues in a variety of these crops resulting from application of alpha-cypermethrin at the recommended rate ranged between 0.05 and 1.0 mg/kg (Shell, 1984). In comparison, residues of cypermethrin in crops were higher and ranged between 0.05 and 2.0 mg/kg. In comparative trials where alpha-cypermethrin was applied at half the dose rate of cypermethrin, alpha-cypermethrin residues in general averaged 40% (20-50%) of those in cypermethrin-treated samples (Shell, 1984; WHO, 1989).

The residue data on cypermethrin have been evaluated by the Joint FAO/WHO Meeting on Pesticide Residues and recommended MRLs (1979/1981) have been published (FAO/WHO, 1980, 1982) (see Table 10). From the available residue data obtained with good agricultural practice and using the MRLs set for cypermethrin, suggested MRLs for alpha-cypermethrin can be extrapolated (Table 10).

It can be concluded that alpha-cypermethrin, since it is biologically more active, is always used at a lower application rate than cypermethrin and, as a result, the residues on crops are approximately half those of cypermethrin.

Table 10. Comparison of current MRLs in mg/kg product for cypermethrin recommended by the FAO/WHO Joint Meeting on Pesticides Residues (JMPR) with those which may be proposed for alpha-cypermethrin

Commodity	Cypermethrin (JMPR)[a]	Alpha-cypermethrin (extrapolated)
Cotton seed	0.2	0.05
Rapeseed	0.2	0.05
Pome fruits	2	0.5
Peaches	2	0.5
Grapes	1	0.5
Citrus fruits	2	1
Tomatoes	0.5	0.1
Brassica, leafy vegetables	1	1
Lettuce	2	1
Peas, kidney beans (less pod)	0.05	0.05
Soyabeans (less pod)	0.05	0.05
Potatoes	0.05	0.05
Sugarbeet (roots)	0.05	0.05
Maize grain	0.05	0.05

[a] From: FAO/WHO (1980, 1982)
For analytical reasons, 0.05 mg/kg is considered the minimum practical MRL.

10.2 Environmental impact

Because its physico-chemical properties are similar to those of cypermethrin, alpha-cypermethrin is expected to have a similar environmental fate to that of cypermethrin. The potential of alpha-cypermethrin to bioaccumulate may therefore be estimated from experimental data on the bioaccumulation of cypermethrin. This is because the octanol/water partition coefficients of alpha-cypermethrin (1.4×10^5; log $P_{ow} = 5.16$) and cypermethrin (2×10^6; log $P_{ow} = 6.3$) are relatively similar. In fish, the bioaccumulation of cypermethrin determined experimentally was lower than might have been expected from its partition coefficient, presumably because it was rapidly metabolized. This would also be expected for alpha-cypermethrin because both the route of metabolism and its rate are similar to those of cypermethrin (Shell, 1983b; WHO, 1989).

In the area of environmental toxicology, results available for green algae, aquatic invertebrates, fish and bees show that the acute toxicity of alpha-cypermethrin is slightly higher than, but broadly similar to that of cypermethrin (Table 11). This is because the toxicity of cypermethrin results largely from its alpha-cypermethrin component. No toxicity data are available concerning the effects of alpha-cypermethrin on soil microbes, but little or no effect on carbon dioxide evolution, oxygen uptake and nitrogen fixation would be expected if alpha-cypermethrin acts on soil microbes in a similar way to cypermethrin (WHO, 1989). There are also no toxicity data for alpha-cypermethrin in birds. However, cypermethrin has a low toxicity to birds. Since alpha-cypermethrin constitutes 25% of the active ingredients of cypermethrin and is used at lower application rates, it is expected that alpha-cypermethrin will also have a low toxicity to birds (Shell, 1983b).

Overall, in the natural environment, the more biologically active alpha-cypermethrin is likely to have a similar toxicity to that of cypermethrin. This is because alpha-cypermethrin is used at a lower application rate than cypermethrin.

10.3 Mammalian toxicity

In acute oral toxicity studies, alpha-cypermethrin is either equally toxic or two to three times more toxic than cypermethrin (WHO, 1989), depending on the vehicle and the concentrations used.

In Table 12, the no-observed-effect levels and lowest-observed-effect levels of the various mouse, rat and dog studies are compared for cypermethrin, *cis*-cypermethrin and alpha-cypermethrin. Short- and long-term studies with the racemic mixture cypermethrin (containing four cis and four trans isomers), *cis*-cypermethrin (four cis isomers) and alpha-cypermethrin (two cis isomers) have shown similar toxicological effects.

The data from the short-term toxicity studies indicate that alpha-cypermethrin is approximately 2 to 3 times more toxic than cypermethrin in rats and dogs. This reflects the amount of alpha-cypermethrin present in cypermethrin.

The signs of intoxication, the effects on target organs and tissues, and the metabolic pathway of alpha-cypermethrin are similar to those of *cis*-cypermethrin. The mode of action of alpha-cypermethrin is similar to that of cypermethrin.

Table 11. Comparison of environmental toxicology of cypermethrin and alpha-cypermethrin

Species	Life stage/ age	Water temper- ature (°C)	Administration route or vehicle	Measured end-point	Values for cypermethrin	Values for alpha-cypermethrin	Reference
Green alga							
(*Selenastrum capricornutum*)	-	24	dispersal via acetone	2- to 4-day EC_{50} (growth)	> 100 μg/litre	> 100 μg/litre	Stephenson (1982)
Aquatic invertebrates							
Water flea (*Daphnia magna*)	up to 24 h old	20	dispersal via acetone	EC_{50} (immobilization)			Stephenson (1982)
				24 h	1.2 μg/litre	1.1 μg/litre	
				48 h	0.3 μg/litre	0.3 μg/litre	
Fish							
Rainbow trout (*Oncorhynchus mykiss*)	3.3 g	15	dispersal via acetone	96-h LC_{50}	2.8 μg/litre	2.8 μg/litre	Stephenson (1982)
Fathead minnow (*Pimephales promelas*)	0.74-0.76 g (juvenile)	23-25	absorbed on to pumice	96-h LC_{50}	1.2 μg/litre	0.93 μg/litre	Stephenson (1983)
Earthworm							
(*Eisenia foetida*)	-	-	filter paper contact toxicity	48-h LD_{50}	26.1 μg/cm^2	10 μg/cm^2	Roberts & Dorough (1984); Inglesfield & Sherwood (1983)
Bees							
(*Apis mellifera*)	worker	-	oral administration	24-h LD_{50}	0.035 μg/bee	0.06 μg/bee	Badmin & Twydell (1976); Murray (1985)

Table 12. Comparison between short- and long-term oral studies with cypermethrin, *cis*-cypermethrin and alpha-cypermethrin

Animal species	Number of studies	Duration of experiment	Dose level in mg/kg diet No-observed-effect level	Lowest-observed-effect level
Cypermethrin (4 cis and 4 trans isomers)[a]				
Mouse	1	2 years	400	1600
Rat	1	5 weeks	750	1500
	2	13 weeks	100/150	400
	1	2 years	100	1000
Dog	1	13 weeks	500	1500
	1	2 years	300	750/600
***cis*-cypermethrin (4 cis isomers)**[a]				
Rat	1	5 weeks	100	300
Alpha-cypermethrin (2 cis isomers)				
Rat	1	5 weeks	200	400
	1	13 weeks	60	180
Dog	2	2-7 days	200	250
	1	13 weeks	90	270

[a] See WHO (1989)

Cypermethrin has been tested in a rodent multigeneration reproduction study and for embryotoxicity and teratogenicity in two species. There were no effects on either reproductive performance or on fetal development, even at doses producing systemic toxicity (WHO, 1989). Alpha-cypermethrin has not been tested for reproductive toxicity or teratogenicity, but there is no indication that it would have effects on these parameters since it is a component of cypermethrin.

The WHO Task Group on Environmental Health Criteria for Cypermethrin, which met in 1986, concluded that cypermethrin was without mutagenic activity. Available data on alpha-cypermethrin indicate that this compound also is non-mutagenic in tests with *Salmonella typhimurium*, *Saccharomyces cerevisiae*, and *in vivo* and *in vitro* tests with rat liver cells for the induction of chromosome aberration and production of DNA single-strand damage.

Alpha-cypermethrin has not been tested for carcinogenicity, but the long-term toxicity studies in mice and rats did not indicate any carcinogenic potential for cypermethrin. Because cypermethrin contains the two cis isomers present in alpha-cypermethrin, it is unlikely that these two isomers would have a carcinogenic potential. This supposition is supported by the fact that all the mutagenicity studies on alpha-cypermethrin have yielded negative results.

Near lethal doses of alpha-cypermethrin and cypermethrin produce sparse axonopathy in the peripheral nerves of rats (see section 7.7.2). Similar signs of intoxication were observed with both compounds, and increases in beta-glucuronidase and beta-galactosidase activities, consistent with an axonal degeneration, could only be detected in severely intoxicated animals. The magnitude of the enzyme changes was substantially less than for other known neurotoxic compounds, thereby confirming the minor nature of the lesion. The short time period needed to produce ataxia and/or abnormal gait rules out a causal relationship between ataxia and axonopathy. The signs of intoxication are consistent with a pharmacologically-mediated effect. No biochemical changes indicative of axonopathy were detected in rats given 20 oral doses of 20 mg alpha-cypermethrin/kg body weight per day or 75 mg cypermethrin/kg body weight per day. From these comparative studies, it is clear that the neurotoxic potential of alpha-cypermethrin and cypermethrin is qualitatively similar, but alpha-cypermethrin is 3 to 4 times more potent. This reflects the fact that alpha-cypermethrin constitutes the active ingredient and 25% of cypermethrin.

Appraisal

The effects of alpha-cypermethrin on vertebrates and invertebrates are qualitatively and, in a number of cases, even quantitatively similar to those of cypermethrin, reflecting the fact that alpha-cypermethrin is composed of two of the four cis isomers present in cypermethrin (these two being the most active components of cypermethrin). Therefore, the toxicological information of cypermethrin can be used to evaluate the effects of alpha-cypermethrin where certain important toxicity studies for alpha-cypermethrin are lacking.

Alpha-cypermethrin has a higher toxicity (lower no-observed-effect level) than cypermethrin but its application rate is at most only half that of cypermethrin (5-30 g active ingredient/ha for alpha-cypermethrin and 10-200 g active ingredient/ha for cypermethrin). Therefore, residue levels of alpha-cypermethrin in crops are less than half those of cypermethrin.

11. PREVIOUS EVALUATIONS BY INTERNATIONAL BODIES

The toxicological and residue data on cypermethrin have been evaluated by the Joint FAO/WHO Meeting on Pesticide Residues (JMPR) (FAO/WHO, 1980, 1982), but alpha-cypermethrin has not yet been evaluated by the JMPR.

REFERENCES[a]

Aldridge WN (1990) An assessment of the toxicological properties of pyrethroids and their neurotoxicity. Crit Rev Toxicol, **21**(2): 89-104.

Armitage GD (1984) Fastac exposure study. Analysis of atmospheric and surface wipe samples ex. Durban, South Africa. Sittingbourne, Shell Research (SBRN 84.091).

Badmin JS & Twydell RS (1976) Evaluation of the insecticide WL 43467 against the honey bee *Apis mellifera*. Sittingbourne, Shell Research (WKSR.0021.76).

Baldwin MK (1990) Alpha-cypermethrin (Fastac): Water solubility at various pH values. London, Shell International Chemical Company, Ltd (Internal report SBGR 90.158).

Blair D (1984) The toxicology of pyrethroids; the acute 4-h inhalation toxicity of a 30% m/m Fastac on silica powder formulation. Sittingbourne, Shell Research (SBGR 84.066).

Bosio PG (1982) Study of isomer conversion of WL85871 in various crops from 1981 treatments. Berre, France, Shell Chimie (BEGR 82.031).

Brooks TM (1982) Toxicity studies with pyrethroids; *in vitro* genotoxicity studies with WL85871. Sittingbourne, Shell Research (SBGR 81.273).

Brooks TM (1984) Genotoxicity studies with Fastac; the induction of gene mutation in the yeast *Saccharomyces cerevisiaee* XV 185-14-C. Sittingbourne, Shell Research (SBGR 84.117).

Brown K (1989) A study of the effects on honey-bees of a large scale commercial application of "Fastac" to oilseed rape. London, Shell International Chemical Company, Ltd (Internal report SBGR 89.198).

Clare MG & Wiggins DE (1984) Genotoxicity studies with Fastac; *in vivo* cytogenetic test using rat bone marrow. Sittingbourne, Shell Research (SBGR 84.120).

Clark DG (1982) WL85871; a 90-day feeding study in rats. Sittingbourne, Shell Research, vol 1 and 2 (SBGR 81.293).

Coveney PC & Forbes S (1986) Analysis of soil from UK (Coates) for residues of "Fastac" (WL85871) - soil persistence trial - third year. Sittingbourne, Shell Research (SBGR 86.201).

Creedy CL & Logan CJ (1984) *In vitro* metabolism of cypermethrin isomers by rat, rabbit, and human liver preparations. Sittingbourne, Shell Research (SBGR 84.108).

Dewar AJ (1981) Toxicology of pyrethroids; the acute oral and percutaneous toxicity, skin and eye irritancy and skin sensitizing potential of WL85871 including a comparison with the acute toxicity of WL 43467 (Ripcord). Sittingbourne, Shell Research (TLGR 80.148).

Eadsforth CV, Bragt PC, & Van Sittert NJ (1988) Human dose-excretion studies with pyrethroid insecticides cypermethrin and alpha-cypermethrin; relevance for biological monitoring. Xenobiotica, **18**(5): 603-614.

[a] The proprietary Shell Research reports in the following list were submitted to the IPCS by Shell.

FAO (1982) Second Government Consultation on International Harmonization of Pesticide Registration Requirements, Rome, 11-15 October 1982. Rome, Food and Agriculture Organization of the United Nations.

FAO/WHO (1980) 1979 Evaluations of some pesticide residues in food. Rome, Food and Agriculture Organization of the United Nations (FAO Plant Production and Protection Paper 20 sup).

FAO/WHO (1982) 1981 Evaluations of some pesticide residues in food. Rome, Food and Agriculture Organization of the United Nations (FAO Plant Production and Protection Paper 42).

Fisher JR, Robinson J, & Debray PH (1983) A new multipurpose insecticide. Proceedings of 10th International Congress of Plant Protection, Brighton, England, 20-25 November 1983. Vol. 1, pp 452-459.

Forbes S (1985) Residues of Fastac (WL85871) in cured marine catfish (*Arius* sp.) from Indonesia. Sittingbourne, Shell Research (SBGR 85.200).

Forbes S & Burden AN (1984) Analysis of soil from UK (Reculver) for residues of WL85871 (Fastac) - soil persistence trial - second year. Sittingbourne, Shell Research (SBGR 84.005).

Forbes S & Cole DA (1986) Residues of Fastac (WL85871) in sweetcorn from Canada. Sittingbourne, Shell Research (SBGR 86.217).

Forbes S & Knight CJ (1983) Analysis of soil from UK (Reculver) for residues of WL85871 - soil persistence trial - first year. Sittingbourne, Shell Research (SBGR.83.162).

Forbes S & Mackay CE (1983) Analysis of soil from UK (Coates) for residues of WL85871 (Fastac) - soil persistence trial - first year. Sittingbourne, Shell Research (SBGR 83.418).

Forbes S & Wales GH (1985a) Analysis of soil from UK (Reculver) for residues of Fastac (WL85871) - soil persistence trial - third year. Sittingbourne, Shell Research (SBGR 85.070).

Forbes S & Wales GH (1985b) Analysis of soil from UK (Coates) for residues of Fastac (WL85871) - soil persistence trial - second year. Sittingbourne, Shell Research (SBGR 85.071).

Francis WP & Gill JP (1991) Flufenoxuron/alpha-cypermethrin - residues in sheep tissues following treatment with PAMPASS/RENEGADE mixtures by dip or pour-on. London, Shell International Chemical Company, Ltd (Internal report SBGR 89.254).

Gardner JR (1989) "Fastac/Azodrin" 20/400 g/litre emulsifiable concentrate: Acute oral and dermal toxicity. London, Shell International Chemical Company, Ltd (Internal report SBGR 89.026).

Gardner JR (1991) Fastac 60 G/l SC (SF07396); acute oral and dermal toxicity in rat. Sittingbourne, Shell Research (SBGR 91.020).

Garforth BM (1982a) A comparison of the toxicities of WL85871 and Ripcord to freshwater invertebrates in small field enclosures. Sittingbourne, Shell Research (SBGR 82.015).

Garforth BM (1982b) WL85871 and cypermethrin; chronic toxicity to *Daphnia magna*. Sittingbourne, Shell Research (SBGR 82.119).

Garforth BM & Woodbridge AP (1984) Spray drift from an aerial application of Fastac; fate and biological effects in an adjacent freshwater ditch. Sittingbourne, Shell Research (SBGR 84.055).

Greenough RJ & Goburdhun R (1984) WL85871; Oral (dietary) maximum tolerated dose study in dogs. Musselburgh, Inveresk Research International (Unpublished report No. 3107, submitted to WHO by Shell Research).

Greenough RJ, Cockrill JB, & Goburdhun R (1984) WL85871; 13-week oral (dietary) toxicity study in dogs. Musselburgh, Inveresk Research International (Unpublished report No. 3197, submitted to WHO by Shell Research).

Hend RW (1983) Toxicology of pyrethroids; skin stimulation studies using guinea-pigs. Sittingbourne, Shell Research (SBGR 83.197).

Hillaby JM (1988) Deposition of pesticide on the orchard floor following a commercial mistblower application to apples. London, Shell International Chemical Company, Ltd (Internal report SBGR 88.106).

Hillaby JM & Inglesfield C (1986) The residual toxicity of "Fastac" formulations and "Fastac"/fungicide mixtures to the honey bee, *Apis mellifera* L. Sittingbourne, Shell Research (SBGR 86.018).

Hutson DH (1982) WL85871; metabolism of a single oral dose in the rat. Sittingbourne, Shell Research (SBGR 82.205).

Hutson DH & Logan CJ (1986) The metabolic fate in rats of the pyrethroid insecticide WL85871, a mixture of two isomers of cypermethrin. Pestic Sci, **17**: 548-558.

Inglesfield C (1984) The effects of two formulations of Fastac on the beneficial arthropod fauna of grape vines. Sittingbourne, Shell Research (SBGR 84.039).

Inglesfield C (1985a) A field study on the effects of Fastac on the beneficial arthropod fauna of maize in France. Sittingbourne, Shell Research (SBGR 85.069).

Inglesfield C (1985b) A pond enclosure study of the effects of Fastac formulations on aquatic invertebrates. Sittingbourne, Shell Research (SBGR 85.083).

Inglesfield C (1985c) The effects of the pyrethroid insecticide WL85871 on non-target arthropods: Field studies. Pestic Sci, **16**(2): 211.

Inglesfield C (1988) Effects of "Fastac" on non-target arthropods; an overview of a five-year arable crop rotation study. Sittingbourne, Shell Research (SBGR 87.149).

Inglesfield C (1989) A long-term field study to investigate the effects of alpha-cypermethrin on predatory and parasitic arthropods. Meded Fac Landbouwwet Rijksuniv Gent, **54**(3a): 895-904.

Inglesfield C (1991) Effects of alpha-cypermethrin (Fastac) on entomophagous organisms and game-bird chick-food insects in summer cereals. The Hague, Shell Internationale Petroleum Maatschappij B.V. (Report Series HSE 91.008).

Inglesfield C & Forbes S (1986) A field trial to assess the effects of "Fastac" 100 g/litre OSC on foraging honey bees in oilseed rape. Sittingbourne, Shell Research (SBGR 86.087).

Inglesfield C & Sherwood CM (1983) Toxicity of cypermethrin and WL85871 to the earthworm, *Eisenia foetida* L. (*Oligochaeta:Lumbriculidae*) in laboratory tests. Sittingbourne, Shell Research (SBGR 83.071).

Langner EJ (1980) Determination of the vapour pressure of WL 43467 and WL 85871 at 20 °C. Sittingbourne Shell Research (Research Note No. FCDN 80.137).

Le Blanc J (1985) Field experiments on the effects of a new pyrethroid insecticide WL85871 on bees foraging artificial aphid honey-dew on winter wheat. Pestic Sci, **16**(2): 206.

Le Quesne PM, Maxwell IC, & Butterworth STG (1980) Transient facial sensory symptoms following exposure to synthetic pyrethroids; a clinical and electrophysiological assessment. Neurotoxicology, **2**: 1-11.

Logan CJ (1983) WL85871; depletion from tissues of female rats after a single oral dose. Sittingbourne, Shell Research (SBGR 83.075).

McMinn AL (1983a) The degradation of the pyrethroid insecticides WL85871 (Fastac) and WL43481 in cabbage. Sittingbourne, Shell Research (SBGR 83.396).

McMinn AL (1983b) The degradation of the pyrethroid insecticides WL85871 and WL43481 in soil. Sittingbourne, Shell Research (SBGR 83.395).

Maloney SE, Maule A, & Smith ARW (1988) Microbial transformation of the pyrethroid insecticides: Permethrin, deltamethrin, fastac, fenvalerate and fluvalinate. Appl Environ Microbiol, **54**(11): 2874-2876.

Murray A (1985) Acute and residual toxicity of a new pyrethroid insecticide WL85871, to honey-bees. Bull Environ Contam Toxicol, **34**: 560-564.

Pearson N (1986) Fastac oil-enriched suspension concentrates; acute toxicities of two formulations to the rainbow trout, *Salmo gairdneri*. Sittingbourne, Shell Research (SBGR 85.290).

Pearson N (1990) The fate of "Fastac" in experimental ponds. Sittingbourne, Shell Research (SBGR 88.177).

Pickering RG (1982) A 5-week feeding study with WL85871 in rats. Sittingbourne, Shell Research, vol 1 and 2 (SBGR 81.212).

Price JB (1985a) Toxicology of Fastac (WL85871); the acute oral and percutaneous toxicity and skin irritancy of a Fastac 10% EC (SF 06510). Sittingbourne, Shell Research (SBGR 85.087).

Price JB (1985b) Toxicology of pyrethroids; the acute oral and percutaneous toxicity, skin and eye irritancy of a Fastac 100 g/litre suspension concentrate (SF 06378). Sittingbourne, Shell Research (SBGR 84.298).

Price JB (1986) Toxicology of pyrethroids; the acute oral and percutaneous toxicity, skin and eye irritancy of SF 06615, a 15 g/litre suspension concentrate of WL85871 ("Fastac", "Fendona"). Sittingbourne, Shell Research (SBGR 85.224).

Price JB (1987) Toxicology of pyrethroids; the acute oral and percutaneous toxicity of Fastac/BPMC 10/400 g/litre EC (SF 06717). Sittingbourne, Shell Research (SBGR 86.253).

Price JB (1988) Toxicology of animal health products; the acute oral and percutaneous toxicity, skin and eye irritancy of two pour-on formulations of Renegade, SF 06954 (10 g/litre) and SF 06977 (15 g/litre). Sittingbourne, Shell Research (SBGR 87.161).

Roberts BL & Dorough HW (1984) Relative toxicities of chemicals to the earthworm *Eisenia foedita*. Environ Toxicol Chem, 3(1): 67-68.

Rose GP (1982) Toxicology of pyrethroids; the acute oral and percutaneous toxicity of WL85871 (*cis*-2-Ripcord) comparison with Ripcord. Sittingbourne, Shell Research (SBGR 82.130).

Rose GP (1983a) Toxicology of pyrethroids; the acute oral toxicity of WL85871 in comparison with WL43467. Sittingbourne, Shell Research (SBGR 83.101).

Rose GP (1983b) Neurotoxicity of WL85871 in comparison with WL43467; the effect of twenty oral doses of WL85871 or WL43467 over a period of 4 weeks on the rat sciatic/posterior tibial nerve, trigeminal nerve and trigeminal ganglion. Sittingbourne, Shell Research (SBGR 83.185).

Rose GP (1984a) Toxicology of pyrethroids; the acute intraperitoneal toxicity of technical Fastac. Sittingbourne, Shell Research (SBGR 84.085).

Rose GP (1984b) Toxicology of Fastac; the eye irritancy potential of the Fastac 100 g/litre emulsifiable concentrate formulation DF 05898 and its formulation components. Sittingbourne, Shell Research (SBGR 84.053).

Rose GP (1984c) Toxicology of pyrethroids; the acute oral and percutaneous toxicity, skin and eye irritancy of the Fastac 15 g/litre ULV formulation SF 06363. Sittingbourne, Shell Research (SBGR 84.145).

Rose GP (1984d) Toxicology of pyrethroids; the acute oral and percutaneous toxicity, skin and eye irritancy of the Fastac 10 EC formulation, 5835 B. Sittingbourne, Shell Research (SBGR 84.077).

Rose GP (1984e) Toxicology of pyrethroids; the acute oral and percutaneous toxicity, skin and eye irritancy of the Fastac 10 EC formulation 5898 B. Sittingbourne, Shell Research (SBGR 84.078).

Rose GP (1984f) Toxicology of pyrethroids; the acute oral and percutaneous toxicity, skin and eye irritancy of the Fastac 3 EC formulation, DF 06353. Sittingbourne, Shell Research (SBGR 84.084).

Rose GP (1984g) Toxicology of pyrethroids; the eye irritancy and skin sensitizing potential of the 100 g/litre Fastac emulsifiable concentrate formulation EF 5835. Sittingbourne, Shell Research (SBGR 84.086).

Rose GP (1984h) Toxicology of pyrethroids; the acute oral and percutaneous toxicity, skin and eye irritancy of the 15:120 g/litre Fastac/methomyl emulsifiable concentrate formulation, FD 9148. Sittingbourne, Shell Research (SBGR 84.104).

Rose GP (1985) Toxicology of insecticides; the acute oral and percutaneous toxicity, skin and eye irritancy of the 30 g/litre Fastac EC formulation SF 06446. Sittingbourne, Shell Research (SBGR 84.209).

Senior PL & Lavers A (1990a) Fastac - Potential dermal exposure. The Hague, Shell Internationale Petroleum Maatschappij B.V. (Report Series HSE 90.016).

Senior PL & Lavers A (1990b) A field study of operator exposure to Fastac during crop spraying at Shell Research Ltd, Sittingbourne Research Centre. The Hague, Shell Internationale Petroleum Maatschappij B.V. (Report Series HSE 90.014).

SHELL (1983a) Review of mammalian and human toxicology; Fastac. The Hague, Shell Internationale Petroleum Maatschappij B.V. (Review Series MDT 83.001).

SHELL (1983b) Review of environmental toxicology; Fastac. The Hague, Shell Internationale Petroleum Maatschappij B.V. (Review Series MDT 83.005).

SHELL (1984) Review of residue information; Fastac. London, Shell International Chemical Company Ltd.

SHELL (1986) Determination of residues of alpha-cypermethrin in rat blood - Gas chromatographic method. Sittingbourne, Shell Research (Analytical Method Series, No. SAMS 436-1).

SHELL (1987a) Determination of WL 85871 and the ratio of the enantiomer pairs in technical material and formulated products - liquid chromatographic method. Sittingbourne, Shell Research (Analytical Methods Series, No. SAMS 346-4).

SHELL (1987b) Intereg residues section: Ripcord residues in crops. London, International Chemical Company, Ltd (Internal report).

SHELL (1987c) Intereg residues section: Fastac residues in crops. London, International Chemical Company, Ltd (Internal report).

SHELL (1988a) Determination of residues of alpha-cypermethrin in animal tissues - Gas-liquid chromatographic method. Sittingbourne, Shell Research (Analytical Method Series, No. SAMS 461-1).

SHELL (1988b) Determination of residues of alpha-cypermethrin in milk - Gas-liquid chromatographic method. Sittingbourne, Shell Research (Analytical Method Series, No. SAMS 456-1).

SHELL (1989a) Determination of residues of alpha-cypermethrin in crops - Gas chromatographic method. Sittingbourne, Shell Research (Analytical Method Series, No. SAMS 351-2).

SHELL (1989b) Review of environmental toxicology; Fastac. The Hague, Shell Internationale Petroleum Maatschappij B.V. (Review Series HSE 89.008).

SHELL (1990a) Determination of residues of alpha-cypermethrin in water - Gas chromatographic method. Sittingbourne, Shell Research (Analytical Method Series, No. SAMS 469-2).

SHELL (1990b) Determination of residues of alpha-cypermethrin in soils - Gas chromatographic method. Sittingbourne, Shell Research (Analytical Method Series, No. SAMS 354-2).

Sherren AJ (1988a) Residues of alpha-cypermethrin in cattle tissues following topical treatment of calves with "Renegade" pour-on in the UK. London, Shell International Chemical Company, Ltd (Internal report SBGR 88.036).

Sherren AJ (1988b) Residues of alpha-cypermethrin in milk following topical treatment of cows with "Renegade" pour-on in the UK. London, Shell International Chemical Company, Ltd (Internal report SBGR 88.037).

Shires SW (1982) A comparison of the toxicity of WL85871 and Ripcord to rainbow trout (*Salmo gairdneri*, Richardson) in small field enclosures. Sittingbourne, Shell Research (SBGR 82.089).

Shires SW (1983a) Pesticides and honey bees; case studies with Ripcord and Fastac. Span, **26**(3): 118-120.

Shires SW (1983b) Effect of formulation type on the toxicity of insecticides to fish. Sittingbourne, Shell Research (SBGR 83.015).

Shires SW (1985a) A step-wise evaluation of the effects of a new pyrethroid insecticide WL85871 on honey bees. Pestic Sci, **16**(2): 205-216.

Shires SW (1985b) Toxicity of a new pyrethroid insecticide WL85871 to rainbow trout. Bull Environ Contam Toxicol, **34**: 134-137.

Shires SW & Inglesfield C (1986) A field study of the effects of "Fastac" (WL85871) on rice pests and their natural enemies. Sittingbourne, Shell Research (SBGR 86.003).

Shires SW, Le Blanc J, Debray P, Forbes S, & Louveaux J (1984a) Field experiments on the effects of a new pyrethroid insecticide WL85871 on bees foraging artificial aphid honey-dew on winter wheat. Pestic Sci, **15**: 543-552.

Shires SW, Murray A, Debray P, & Le Blanc J (1984b) The effects of a new pyrethroid insecticide WL85871 on foraging honey bees (*Apis mellifera* L.) Pestic Sci, **15**: 491-499.

Shires SW, Le Blanc J, Murray A, Forbes S, & Debray P (1984c) A field trial to assess the effects of a new pyrethroid insecticide WL85871 on foraging honey bees in oilseed rape. J Agric Res, **23**(4): 217-226.

Stephenson RR (1982) WL85871 and cypermethrin; a comparison of their acute toxicity to *Salmo gairdneri, Daphnia magna* and *Selenastrum capricornutum*. Sittingbourne, Shell Research (SBGR 81.277).

Stephenson RR (1983) WL85871 and cypermethrin; a comparative study of their toxicity to the fathead minnow, *Pimephales promelas* (Rafinesque). Sittingbourne, Shell Research (SBGR 82.298).

Stephenson RR (1986) "Fastac"; the acute toxicity of different formulations to fish in rice paddies. Sittingbourne, Shell Research (SBGR 85.201).

Stephenson RR (1987a) The effects of "Fastac" (OSC) on fish survival and growth following its application to paddy rice. Sittingbourne, Shell Research (SBGR 87.054).

Stephenson RR (1987b) An insecticide formulation that spares fish. Span, **30**(2): 75-77.

Stephenson RR (1987c) The effects of "Fastac" (OSC) on fish following its application to outdoor tanks. Sittingbourne, Shell Research (SBGR 86.227).

Stone CM & Watkinson RJ (1983) WL85871; an assessment of ready biodegradability. Sittingbourne, Shell Research (SBGR 83.206).

Tasei J-N, Carre S, Bosio PG, Debray P, & Hariot J (1987) Effects of the pyrethroid insecticide WL85871 and Phosalone on adults and progeny of the leaf-cutting bee, *Megachile rotundata* F., pollinator of lucerne. Pestic Sci, **21**: 119-128.

Van Sittert NJ, Eadsforth CV, & Bragt P (1985) Human oral dose-excretion study with Fastac. The Hague, Shell Internationale Petroleum Maatschappij B.V. (Report Series HSE 85.010).

Vijverberg HPM & Van Den Bercken J (1990) Neurotoxicological effects and the mode of action of pyrethroid insecticides. Crit Rev Toxicol, **21**(2): 105-126.

Western NJ (1984) Report on the assessment of Fastac exposures during formulation of technical concentrate (TC) and technical material (TM) at Durban, South Africa, September 1983. The Hague, Shell Internationale Petroleum Maatschappij B.V. (Report Series HSE 84.003).

WHO (1989) Environmental Health Criteria 82: Cypermethrin. Geneva, World Health Organization, 154 pp.

Wooder MF (1982) Studies on the effect of WL85871 on the integrity of rat liver DNA *in vivo*. Sittingbourne, Shell Research (SBGR 81.225).

Woollen BH, Marsh JR, & Chester G (1991) Metabolite profiles of a pyrethroid insecticide following oral and dermal absorption in man. In: Proceedings of a Conference on Percutaneous Penetration, Southampton, England, 10-12 April 1991.

Worthing CR & Hance RJ (1991) Fastac. In: The pesticides manual: a world compendium, 9th ed. Croydon, British Crop Protection Council, pp 210-211.

APPENDIX I

Cypermethrin: Summary, Evaluation, Conclusions, and Recommendations (Reprint from EHC 82 on Cypermethrin, WHO/IPCS, 1989)

1. Summary

1.1 General

Cypermethrin was initially synthesized in 1974 and first marketed in 1977 as a highly active synthetic pyrethroid insecticide, effective against a wide range of pests in agriculture, public health, and animal husbandry. In agriculture, its main use is against foliage pests and certain surface soil pests, such as cutworms, but because of its rapid breakdown in soil, it is not recommended for use against soil-borne pests below the surface.

In 1980, 92.5% of all the cypermethrin produced in the world was used on cotton; in 1982, world production was 340 tonnes of the active material. It is mainly used in the form of an emulsifiable concentrate, but ultra-low volume concentrates, wettable powders, and combined formulations with other pesticides are also available.

Chemically, cypermethrin is the alpha-cyano-3-phenoxybenzyl ester of the dichloro analogue of chrysanthemic acid, 2,2-dimethyl-3-(2,2-dichlorovinyl)cyclopropanecarboxylic acid. The molecule embodies three chiral centres, two in the cyclopropane ring and one on the alpha cyano carbon. These isomers are commonly grouped into four cis and four trans isomers, the cis group being the more powerful insecticide. The ratio of cis to trans isomers varies from 50:50 to 40:60. Cypermethrin is the racemic mixture of all eight isomers and, in this appraisal, cypermethrin refers exclusively to the racemic mixture (ratio 50:50) unless otherwise stated.

Most technical grades of cypermethrin contain more than 90% of the active material. The material varies in physical form from a brown-yellow viscous liquid to a semi-solid.

Cypermethrin has a very low vapour pressure and solubility in water, but it is highly soluble in a wide range of organic solvents. Analytical methods are available for the determination of cypermethrin in commercially available preparations. In addition, methods for the determination of residues of cypermethrin in foods and in the environment are well established. In most substrates, the practical limit of determination is 0.01 mg/kg.

1.2 Environmental transport, distribution and transformation

Unlike the natural pyrethrins, cypermethrin is relatively stable to sunlight and, though it is probable that photodegradation plays a significant role in the degradation of the product on leaf surfaces and in surface waters, its effects in soils are limited. The most important photodegradation products, 2,2-dimethyl-3-(2,2-dichlorovinyl) cyclopropane carboxylic acid (CPA), 3-phenoxy-benzoic acid (PBA) and, to some extent, the amide of the intact ester, do not differ greatly from those resulting from biological degradation.

Degradation in the soil occurs primarily through cleavage of the ester linkage to give CPA, PBA, and carbon dioxide. Some of the carbon dioxide is formed through the cleavage of both the cyclopropyl and phenyl rings under oxidative conditions. The half-life of cypermethrin in a typical fertile soil is between 2 and 4 weeks.

Cypermethrin is adsorbed very strongly on soil particles, especially in soils containing large amounts of clay or organic matter. Movement in the soil is therefore extremely limited and downward leaching of the parent molecule through the soil does not occur to an appreciable extent under normal conditions of use. The two principal degradation products show, on the scale of Helling, "intermediate mobility".

Cypermethrin is also relatively immobile in surface waters and, when applied to the surface of a body of water at rates typical of those used in agriculture applications, it is largely confined to the surface film and does not reach deeper levels or the sediment in appreciable concentrations. Cypermethrin also degrades readily in natural waters with a typical half-life of about 2 weeks. It is probable that both photochemical and biological processes play a part. It has been shown that spray drift reaching surface waters adjacent to sprayed fields does not result in long-term residues in such waters.

Accumulation studies have shown that cypermethrin is rapidly taken up by fish (accumulation factor approximately 1000); the half-life of residues in rainbow trout was 8 days. In view of the low concentrations of cypermethrin that are likely to arise in water bodies and their rapid decline, it has been concluded that, under practical conditions, residues in fish will not reach measurable levels.

The results of field studies have shown that, when applied at recommended rates, the levels of cypermethrin and its degradation products in soil and surface waters are very low. Thus, it is unlikely that the recommended use of cypermethrin will have any effects on the environment.

1.3 Environmental levels and human exposure

Cypermethrin is used in a wide range of crops. In general, the maximum residue limits are low, ranging from 0.05 to 2.0 mg/kg in the different food commodities. The residues will be further reduced during food processing. In food of animal origin, residues may range between 0.01 and 0.2 mg/kg product. Residues in non-food commodities are generally higher, ranging up to 20 mg/kg product.

Total dietary intake values for man are not available, but it can be expected that the oral exposure of the general population is low to negligible.

1.4 Kinetics and metabolism

Absorption of cypermethrin from the gastrointestinal tract and its elimination are quite rapid. The major metabolic reaction is cleavage of the ester bond. Elimination of the cyclopropane moiety in the rat, over a 7-day period, ranged from 40 to 60% in the urine and from 30 to 50% in the faeces; elimination of the phenoxybenzyl moiety was about 30% in the urine and 55 to 60% in the faeces. Biliary excretion is a minor route of elimination for the cyclopropane moiety and small amounts are exhaled as carbon dioxide. In principle, these absorption and elimination rates and metabolic pathways hold for all animal species studied, including domestic animals. In cows fed 100 mg cypermethrin/day, the highest level found in milk was 0.03 mg/litre; levels of up to 0.1 mg/kg tissue were found in subcutaneous fat. Under practical conditions, the oral intake of cypermethrin with feed will be much lower. Cypermethrin used as a spray or dip to combat parasites, may give rise to maximum residues of 0.05 mg/kg tissue and 0.01 mg/litre milk.

Laying hens exposed orally to 10 mg cypermethrin/kg diet for 2 weeks, showed cypermethrin levels of up to 0.1 mg/kg in the fat, and up to 0.09 mg/kg in the eggs (predominantly in the yolk).

Consistent with the lipophilic nature of cypermethrin, the highest mean tissue concentrations are found in body fat, skin, liver, kidneys, adrenals, and ovaries. Only negligible concentrations are found in the brain. The half-life of *cis*-cypermethrin in the fat of the rat ranges from 12 to 19 days and that of the trans isomer, from 3 to 4 days. In mice, these half-lives are 13 days and 1 day, respectively.

Overall, the metabolic transformation has been similar in the different animals studied, including man. Differences that occur have been related to the rate of formation rather than to the nature of the metabolites formed and to conjugation reactions. Cypermethrin (both the cis and trans isomers) is metabolized via the cleavage of the ester bond to phenoxybenzoic acid and cyclopropane carbolic acid. The fact that thiocyanate has been identified in *in vivo* studies, indicates that the cyanide moiety is further metabolized. The 3-phenoxybenzoic acid is mainly excreted as a conjugate. The type of conjugate differs in a number of animal species. Phenoxybenzoic acid is further metabolized to a hydroxy derivative and conjugated with glucuronic acid or sulfate. The cyclopropyl moiety is mainly excreted as a glucuronide conjugate, hydroxylation of the methyl group only occurring to a limited extent.

Ester cleavage is much slower in certain fish species than in other animal species, the main metabolic pathway being hydroxylation of the phenoxybenzoic and the cyclopropyl moieties.

Ester cleavage also takes place in plants. The phenoxybenzyl and cyclopropyl moieties are readily converted into glucoside conjugates. In mammals, these conjugates are hydrolysed into the original acids and metabolized.

1.5 Effects on organisms in the environment

High doses of cypermethrin may exert transient minor effects on microflora activity in the soil. However, no influence on ammonification and nitrification has been found.

Cypermethrin is very toxic for fish (in laboratory tests 96-h LC_{50}s were generally within the range of 0.4-2.8 μg/litre), and aquatic invertebrates (LC_{50}s in the range of 0.01 - > 5 μg/litre). The presence of suspended solids decreases the toxicity by at least a factor of 2, because of adsorption of cypermethrin to the solids.

Cypermethrin is not very toxic for birds. Signs of cypermethrin intoxication were seen at dose levels of 3000 mg/kg body weight or more. Administration of 1000 mg cypermethrin/kg body weight to laying hens over a 5-day period did not cause signs of intoxication. However, cypermethrin was highly toxic for honey bees in laboratory tests, the oral LD_{50} ranging from 0.03 to 0.12 μg/bee. Under field conditions, the hazard is considerably lower, because of the repellent effect of cypermethrin on worker honey bees, which lasts for at least 6 h after spraying.

Earthworms are not sensitive to cypermethrin. No deaths occurred in worms exposed to levels of 100 mg/kg soil for 14 days.

In studies involving deliberate overspraying of experimental ponds under field conditions, peak concentrations of 2.6 μg cypermethrin/litre were measured in the water. Fish were not affected, but populations of crustaceae, mites, and surface-breathing insects were severely reduced. Most of these populations returned to normal levels after 15 weeks. Free-swimming dipterous larvae and bottom-dwelling invertebrates, snails, flatworms, etc., were not affected. Under normal agricultural conditions (during which drifts may reach adjacent ditches or streams), the only effects seen in surface-breathing or surface-dwelling insects were hyperactivity or immobilization. The relative toxicity of cypermethrin for pests and their parasites and predators is such that the balance between host/prey and parasites/predator may not be adversely affected in the field. However, care should be taken where predatory mites are important in pest management.

1.6 Effects on experimental animals and in vitro test systems

The acute oral toxicity of cypermethrin is moderate. While LD_{50} values differed considerably among animal species depending on the vehicle used and the cis/trans isomeric ratios, the toxic responses in all species were found to be very similar. The acute toxicity of the trans isomer in the rat (LD_{50} > 2000 mg/kg body weight) was lower than that of the cis isomer (LD_{50}, 160-300 mg/kg body weight). The onset of toxic signs of poisoning was rapid and they disappeared within several days in survivors. The toxic signs are characterized by salivation, tremors, increased startle response, sinuous writhing of the whole body (choreoathetosis), and clonic seizures. Myelin and axon degeneration were noted in the sciatic nerve at near lethal dose levels.

Cypermethrin was moderately to severely irritating, when applied to the skin or the eye of the rabbit. The severity was partly dependent on the vehicle used. In guinea-pigs, a mild skin sensitizing potential was found using the maximization test.

No toxic effects were observed in rats, fed cypermethrin at 100 mg/kg diet for 3 months. Furthermore, prolonged feeding of cypermethrin (2 years) to dogs at a level of 300 mg/kg feed did not produce any toxicological effects. A level of 600 mg/kg diet resulted in reduced body weight gain, but no gross pathological or histopathological effects were seen.

Two long-term studies on rats and one on mice were carried out. The dose levels in the rat studies ranged up to 1500 mg/kg diet, equivalent to 75 mg/kg body weight. No effects were seen at 150 mg/kg diet. At the highest dose level, reduced body weight gain, increased liver weights (accompanied by increased smooth endoplasmatic reticulum), and some haematological and biochemical changes were observed. No increase in tumour incidence was noted. The same type of effects were seen in the mouse study at 1600 mg cypermethrin/kg diet. No effects were seen in the 400 mg/kg diet group.

The effect of cypermethrin on the immune system was studied in rats. The results showed the possibility of immune suppression by pyrethroids. More attention should be paid to this aspect, but, at present, no opinion can be given about its relevance in the extrapolation of these data for man.

Repeated oral administration of cypermethrin to rats and other animal species at levels sufficiently high to produce significant mortality in one group of animals, produced biochemical changes in the peripheral nerves, consistent with sparse axonal degeneration. Histopathological changes (swelling and/or disintegration of axons of the sciatic nerve) were observed. There was no cumulative effect. The magnitude of the change was substantially less than that encountered with established neurotoxic agents. The neurotoxic effects seem to be reversible; presumably the clinical signs are not related to the induction of neuropathological lesions.

Further evidence to support the minor nature of the nerve lesions has been afforded by electrophysiological studies on rats. Measurements of the maximal motor conduction velocities of the sciatic and tail nerves of rats were made before, and at intervals of up to 5 weeks after, exposure to a single dose or repeated high doses of cypermethrin. It was concluded from the results that, even at near-lethal doses, cypermethrin did not cause any effects on maximal motor conduction velocities and conduction velocities of the slower motor fibres in rat peripheral nerves. No delayed neurotoxicity was observed in domestic hens.

The ability of the major metabolite of cypermethrin, 3-phenoxybenzoic acid, to produce axonal changes has been investigated and found to be negative.

In a multigeneration reproduction study on rats, dose levels up to 500 mg/kg feed were tested. The parent animals at the highest dose level showed decreased food intake and reduction in body weight gain. No influence on reproductive performance or on survival of the offspring was found. However, at the highest dose level, reductions in litter size and total litter weights were seen. The pooled body weights of weaning pups of the 500 mg/kg group were decreased over 3 generations. No effect was found with 100 mg cypermethrin/kg diet.

Embryotoxic and teratogenic effects were not found in rats administered dose levels of up to 70 mg/kg body weight and clear teratogenic effects were not observed in rabbits given dose levels of up to 30 mg/kg body weight during days 6-18 of gestation.

Cypermethrin did not show any mutagenic activity in bacteria or in yeast, with or without metabolic activation, or in V79 Chinese hamster cells. Furthermore, cypermethrin gave negative results in an *in vivo* chromosomal aberration test with Chinese hamsters and in dominant lethal studies on mice. In a host-mediated assay with mice, no increase in the rate of mitotic gene conversion in *Saccharomyces cerevisae* was found. In a chromosome study using the bone marrow cells of Chinese hamsters, cypermethrin did not increase the number of chromosome abnormalities. However, in a micronucleus test with mouse bone marrow cells, an increase in the frequency of polychromatic erythrocytes with micronuclei was found after oral and dermal applications of cypermethrin. Intraperitoneal application gave a negative result. A sister chromatid exchange study using bone marrow cells of mice showed a dose-response related increase in sister chromatid exchanges of dividing cells.

In long-term/carcinogenicity studies, oral administration of cypermethrin to rats did not induce an increase in the incidence of tumours. In a mouse study, dose levels of up to 1600 mg cypermethrin/kg diet did not produce any increase in tumours of types not commonly associated with the mouse strain employed. The incidence of tumours was similar in all groups with the exception of a slight increase in the incidence of benign alveolar lung tumours in the females in the 1600 mg/kg diet group. However, the increased incidence, when compared with concurrent and historical control incidence, was not sufficient to warrant concern. There was no suggestion of increased malignancy and no evidence of a decrease in the latency of the tumours. Furthermore, there was no evidence of a carcinogenic response in the male mice in this study and, as the results of mutagenicity studies on cypermethrin have been mainly negative, it is concluded that there is no evidence for the carcinogenic potential of cypermethrin.

1.7 Mechanism of toxicity

Extensive studies have been carried out to explain the mechanism of toxicity of cypermethrin, especially with regard to the effects on the nervous system. The results strongly suggest that the primary target site of cypermethrin (and of pyrethroid insecticides in general) in the vertebrate nervous system is the sodium channel in the nerve membrane. The alpha-cyano pyrethroids, such as cypermethrin, cause a long-lasting prolongation of the normally transient increase in sodium permeability of the nerve membrane during excitation, resulting in long-lasting trains of repetitive impulses in sense organs and a frequency-dependent depression of the nerve impulse in nerve fibres. Since the mechanisms responsible for nerve impulse generation and conduction are basically the same throughout the entire nervous system, pyrethroids may well act in a similar way in various parts of the central nervous system. It is suggested that the facial skin sensations that may be experienced by people handling cypermethrin are brought about by repetitive firing of sensory nerve terminals in the skin, and may be considered as an early warning signal that exposure has occurred.

1.8 Effects on man

No cases of accidental poisoning have been reported as a result of occupational exposure.

Skin sensations, reported by a number of authors to have occurred during field studies, generally lasted only a few hours and did not persist for more than one day after exposure. Neurological signs were not observed. General medical and extensive clinical blood-chemistry studies, and electrophysiological studies on selected motor and sensory nerves in the legs and arms did not show any abnormalities.

2. Evaluation

Cypermethrin, an alpha-cyano pyrethroid consisting of a mixture of 8 stereoisomers, is a highly active insecticide effective against a wide range of pests in many food and non-food commodities.

It is stable to light and heat, it has a low vapour pressure and is more stable in acidic than in alkaline media. Sensitive analytical methods for the determination of residues in food and the environment are available.

When cypermethrin is applied to crops, residues may occur in soils and surface waters, but biological degradation is fairly rapid and residues do not accumulate in the environment. Photodegradation is unlikely to play an important role. The main route of degradation is cleavage of the ester linkage to give 2 main degradation products containing the cyclopropane, and the phenoxybenzyl moiety. The half-lives in the soil are determined by many factors, but are in the range of 2-4 weeks. Cypermethrin is strongly adsorbed by soil and downward leaching is negligible. Because of its rather fast breakdown forming less toxic products, and the low dose rates used in good agricultural practice, it is unlikely that cypermethrin will attain significant levels in the environment.

Bioaccumulation in certain organisms, such as fish, took place under laboratory conditions, but levels declined on cessation of exposure and there are indications that, under natural conditions, fish will not contain measurable residues.

When applied according to good agricultural practice, the levels of cypermethrin residues in food commodities are generally low. Total diet studies are not available, but from the available residue information, it can be inferred that the oral intake by man is well below the ADI.

High dose levels of cypermethrin may exert transient effects on the soil microflora. Earthworms and other soil organisms are generally rather resistant to cypermethrin, while fish and other aquatic invertebrates are very sensitive. Because of its strong adsorption on soil, only low levels of cypermethrin may leak into surface water. These may have transient effects, mainly on surface breathing insects.

The toxicity of cypermethrin for birds is low. Bees appear to be very sensitive in laboratory tests. Under field conditions, the effect on bees is minimal, because cypermethrin seems to have a repellent effect for bees. Absorption and elimination of cypermethrin has been rapid in the different mammalian species tested. The major metabolic reaction is cleavage of the ester bond followed by hydroxylation and conjugation of the cyclopropane and phenoxybenzyl moiety. The highest levels are found in body fat, which is consistent with the lipophilic nature of cypermethrin. The half-life in the fat of the rat is about 12-19 days for the cis isomer and 3-4 days for the trans isomer. Breakdown products in plants are bound as glucosides.

The acute toxicity of cypermethrin for mammals is of a moderate order. The oral LD_{50} for the rat ranges from 200 to 4000 mg/kg body weight. Short-term and long-term toxicity studies on rats, mice, and dogs have shown effects on growth, on the liver and kidneys, and the nervous system, and on haematology. A no-observed-adverse-effect level of 7.5 mg/kg body weight has been adopted by the Task Group.

Cypermethrin was not carcinogenic for mice or rats fed diets containing high levels of the material over a 2-year period. Cypermethrin did not induce teratogenic effects in either rats at 70 mg/kg body weight or rabbits at 30 mg/kg body weight. It was also shown not to have any effects on reproductive performance during a 3-generation reproduction study in rats administered 100 mg/kg diet. In a variety of mutagenicity studies, cypermethrin was shown to be mainly without mutagenic activity.

The mechanism of the action on the nervous system has been extensively studied. From these studies and the occupational studies available, it seems that the skin sensation seen in workers handling cypermethrin, generally lasts only a few hours and does not persist for more than one day after exposure. Other neurological signs were not observed. These skin sensations can be considered to be an early warning that exposure has occurred and that work practice should be reviewed. Cypermethrin may cause eye irritation and may be a sensitizer for certain persons.

3. Conclusions

It can be concluded that:

General population: When applied according to good agricultural practice, exposure of the general population to cypermethrin is negligible and is unlikely to present a hazard.

Occupational exposure: With reasonable work practices, hygiene measures, and safety precautions, the use of cypermethrin is unlikely to present a hazard to those occupationally exposed to it. The occurrence of "facial sensations" is an indication of exposure. Under these circumstances work practice should be reviewed.

Environment: With recommended application rates it is unlikely that cypermethrin or its degradation products will attain levels of environmental significance. Notwithstanding its high toxicity for fish and honey bees, this is only likely to cause a problem in the case of spillage and overspraying.

4. Recommendations

- Cypermethrin should be included among the residues looked for in surveillance, market-basket, or total diet studies.

- Attention should be paid to the implications for the welfare of human beings of animal studies indicating immune suppression.

- Further follow-up studies into the facial effects in human beings should be conducted, in order to better understand this phenomenon.

RESUME ET EVALUATION; CONCLUSIONS ET RECOMMANDATIONS

1. Résumé et évaluation

1.1 Identité, emploi, destinée et concentrations dans l'environnement

L'alpha-cyperméthrine est constituée à plus de 90% de l'énantiomère le plus actif du point de vue insecticide parmi les quatre isomères cis qui entrent dans la composition de la cyperméthrine racémique.

C'est un pyréthrinoïde extrêmement actif, qui agit contre de nombreux parasites auxquels on a affaire dans l'agriculture et l'élevage. Il est commercialisé sous forme de concentrés émulsionnables, de formulations à très bas volume, de concentrés pour suspension ou en mélange avec d'autres insecticides.

Le produit technique se présente sous la forme d'une poudre cristalline facilement soluble dans l'acétone, la cyclohexanone et le xylène mais peu soluble dans l'eau. Il est stable en milieu acide ou neutre mais s'hydrolyse à pH 12-13. Il se décompose au-dessus de 120 °C.

On ne dispose d'aucune donnée sur la concentration de l'alpha-cyperméthrine dans l'air.

Dans l'eau, il est probable que l'alpha-cyperméthrine est décomposée par voie photochimique et biologique. On a constaté que, après avoir traité un étang à raison de 15 g de matière active par hectare, les eaux de surface et les couches plus profondes contenaient respectivement 5% et 19% de la dose appliquée une journée après l'épandage et 0,1% et 2% respectivement de cette dose sept jours plus tard. Environ 5% de la dose appliquée se retrouvaient dans les sédiments 16 jours après l'épandage.

Il est probable que l'alpha-cyperméthrine est fortement adsorbée aux particules du sol. Une année après un épandage à raison de 0,5 kg de matière active par hectare, on retrouvait dans le sol des résidus inférieurs à 0,1 mg/kg.

Le coefficient de partage de l'alpha-cyperméthrine entre le n-octanol et l'eau est égal à 1,4 x 10^5 (log de P_{ow} = 5,16).

La dose d'emploi recommandée pour l'alpha-cyperméthrine est moindre que pour la cyperméthrine car elle est biologiquement plus active. Il en résulte moins de résidus sur les récoltes et si l'on se conforme aux doses recommandées, ils se situent entre 0,05 et 1 mg/kg. Chez des poissons-chats d'eau de mer traités à raison de 0,01 à 0,05% p/p de matière active, on a mesuré des résidus de 0,3 à 30 mg/kg une semaine après l'entreposage et entre 0,22 et 4,0 mg/kg 15 semaines plus tard.

1.2 Cinétique et métabolisme

Après avoir été administrée par voie orale à des rats, l'alpha-cyperméthrine est éliminée dans les urines sous forme du sulfo-conjugué de l'acide 3-(4-hydroxyphénoxy)benzoïque ainsi que dans les matières fécales, en partie sans modification. Environ 90% d'une dose orale unique sont éliminées de l'organisme en quatre jours, dont 78% au cours du premier jour. Les résidus sont faibles dans les tissus, sauf dans les tissus lipidiques. Trois jours après administration d'une dose orale unique de 2 mg/kg, la concentration dans les graisses était de 0,4 mg/kg. L'élimination à partir des graisses est biphasique; la demi-vie relative à la phase initiale est de 2,5 jours, et de 17 à 26 jours pour la deuxième phase.

L'alpha-cyperméthrine est métabolisée par coupure de la liaison ester. Chez le rat, la fraction alcool phénoxybenzylique est hydroxylée et transformée en sulfo-conjugué; la fraction acide cyclopropane-carboxylique subit également une conjugaison, probablement sous forme de glucuronide, avant d'être excrétée par la voie urinaire. Des études portant sur des microsomes hépatiques de rats, de lapins et d'origine humaine ont montré que chez ces trois espèces, il pouvait y avoir hydrolyse de l'ester et métabolisation oxydative mais que l'hydrolyse de l'ester prédominait dans le cas des préparations de foie provenant de lapins ou de sujets humains.

Chez l'homme, 43% d'une dose orale (0,25-0,75 mg/litre) ont été excrétés dans les 24 heures par la voie urinaire sous forme d'acide *cis*-cyclopropane-carboxylique libre ou conjugué. Après l'administration de cinq doses quotidiennes successives, l'excrétion urinaire n'a pas augmenté.

On a trouvé de fortes concentrations (jusqu'à 1156 mg/kg) d'alpha-cyperméthrine dans la laine de mouton, 14 jours après avoir traité les animaux par des bains ou des aspersions. De faibles quantités ont été retrouvées dans la graisse sous-cutanée (jusqu'à 0,04 mg/kg). Après avoir traité des veaux le long de l'épine dorsale avec 10 ml d'une formulation à 1,6%, on n'a pas retrouvé d'alpha-cyperméthrine dans les muscles ni le foie. La concentration maximale dans la graisse périrénale était de 0,25 mg/kg au bout de 14 jours.

Après avoir traité des vaches en lactation le long de l'épine dorsale avec des formulations contenant jusqu'à 0,2 g de matière active on a retrouvé dans le lait de 3 des 15 animaux traités, des résidus d'alpha-cyperméthrine compris entre 0,003 et 0,005 mg/litre.

1.3 Effets sur les mammifères de laboratoire et les systèmes d'épreuves in vitro

L'alpha-cyperméthrine présente une toxicité orale aiguë modérée à forte pour les rongeurs. La DL_{50} varie beaucoup chez la souris et le rat et dépend de la concentration du composé et du véhicule utilisé. En pratique, on considère qu'une DL_{50} de 80 mg/kg de poids corporel est représentative. Toutefois, on a fait état de valeurs plus élevées pour la DL_{50} par voie orale dans des conditions d'intoxication aiguë. Une intoxication aiguë par voie orale entraîne des signes cliniques qui traduisent une action au niveau du système nerveux central.

Une application cutanée d'alpha-cyperméthrine à des rats et des souris aux doses respectives de 100 et 500 mg/kg de poids corporel, n'a entraîné ni mortalité ni signes d'intoxication. De même, des rats à qui l'on avait fait inhaler pendant quatre heures de l'alpha-cyperméthrine à une concentration de 400 mg/m^3, n'ont présenté aucune mortalité ni signes cliniques d'intoxication.

L'alpha-cyperméthrine technique ne provoquerait qu'une irritation minimale de la peau chez le lapin. En revanche, certaines formulations de ce composé peuvent déterminer une très forte irritation oculaire. L'alpha-cyperméthrine technique n'a pas d'effet sensibilisant cutané. Chez le cobaye, elle provoque une stimulation des terminaisons nerveuses sensorielles de l'épiderme.

Exposés pendant une courte période à de l'alpha-cyperméthrine à des concentrations quotidiennes allant jusqu'à 200 mg/kg de nourriture pendant cinq semaines ou jusqu'à 100 mg/kg de nourriture pendant 13 semaines, des rats n'ont pas présenté d'effets toxiques. Aux doses les plus élevées, on notait des signes d'intoxication traduisant une atteinte du système nerveux, ainsi qu'une réduction de la croissance et une augmentation du poids du foie et des reins. Aucun effet bien net n'a été observé en ce qui concerne les paramètres hématologiques ou histopathologiques.

Lors d'une étude de 13 semaines au cours de laquelle des chiens ont reçu de l'alpha-cyperméthrine par voie orale, on a observé que la dose la plus forte (270 mg/kg de nourriture) produisait des signes d'intoxication; en revanche tous les autres paramètres étudiés (NFS, biochimie du sang, urines, poids des organes, anatomopathologie et histopathologie) sont restés normaux. La dose sans effet observable était de 90 mg/kg de nourriture (soit l'équivalent de 2,25 mg/kg de poids corporel par jour).

Le même genre d'étude menée sur des rats a montré que l'alpha-cyperméthrine provoquait des effets neurotoxiques imputables à des lésions histopathologiques des nerfs tibial et sciatique, une dégénérescence des axones et un accroissement de l'activité de la bêta-galactosidase.

On ne dispose d'aucune donnée sur la toxicité à long terme, la toxicité pour la fonction de reproduction, la tératogénicité ou l'immunotoxicité.

En se basant sur les données disponibles, on peut conclure que l'alpha-cyperméthrine n'est pas mutagène, comme le montrent les tests effectués sur *Salmonella typhimurium*, *Escherichia coli* et *Saccharomyces cerevisiae* ainsi que les épreuves *in vivo* et *in vitro* sur des cellules de foie de rat, qui n'ont révélé ni aberration chromosomique ni lésion de l'ADN monobrin. On n'a pas non plus observé d'augmentation du nombre d'aberrations chromosomiques dans des cellules de moelle osseuse de rat.

On ne dispose d'aucune donnée sur la cancérogénicité de l'alpha-cyperméthrine.

1.4 Effets sur l'homme

Dans la mesure où l'alpha-cyperméthrine est utilisée conformément aux règles de bonne pratique agricole, l'exposition de la population générale reste négligeable. On a constaté que l'exposition professionnelle cutanée des opérateurs procédant à la préparation des mélanges, au chargement des pulvérisateurs, à l'épandage de l'insecticide ou au lavage du matériel, pouvait atteindre des valeurs respectivement égales à 2,94 mg, 0,61 mg et 0,73 mg.

Lors d'une étude sur l'exposition à l'alpha-cyperméthrine au cours de la préparation de formulations à base de cet insecticide, on a évalué les niveaux d'exposition par surveillance personnelle et statique de la concentration atmosphérique de ce composé et dosage de ses métabolites urinaires. Au cours des deux jours pendant lesquels les personnes exposées procédaient à la formulation de concentrés techniques, l'exposition individuelle moyenne dans le groupe a été respectivement de 2,8 et 4,9 mg/m^3, l'exposition individuelle moyenne du groupe au produit technique étant de 50,1 mg/m^3 le troisième jour. On n'a pas pu déceler la présence de métabolites dans les urines (limite de détection 0,02 mg/litre). Au cours de la préparation des diverses formulations, les ouvriers ont fait état de sensations au niveau de l'épiderme mais en précisant qu'elles étaient légères.

Aucune intoxication n'a été signalée.

1.5 Effets sur d'autres organismes au laboratoire et dans leur milieu naturel

La CE_{50} à 48 et 96 heures (pour la croissance) chez une algue d'eau douce, *Selenastrum capricornutum*, dépasse 100 µg/litre.

L'alpha-cyperméthrine est très fortement toxique pour les invertébrés aquatiques. Les valeurs de la CE_{50} à 24 et 48 heures (pour l'immobilisation de la daphnie) sont respectivement égales à 1,0 et 0,3 µg/litre, et celle de la CL_{50} à 24 heures (pour *Gammarus pulex*) est égale à 0,05 µg/litre. L'alpha-cyperméthrine est également très toxique pour un certain nombre d'arthropodes aquatiques mais sa toxicité est moindre pour les mollusques. La toxicité à court terme de ce composé peut être réduite lorsqu'il est présenté sous la forme d'une suspension dans l'huile. Les pertes à l'épandage peuvent provoquer des effets toxiques sur les invertébrés aquatiques, mais comme l'alpha-cyperméthrine disparaît rapidement de l'eau, ceux-ci ont la possibilité de récupérer. L'alpha-cyperméthrine est très fortement toxique pour les poissons. La valeur de la CL_{50} à 96 heures oscille entre 0,7 et 350 µg/litre selon le type de formulation. Les concentrés émulsionnables sont beaucoup plus toxiques que les concentrés en suspension, les poudres mouillables et les formulations micro-encapsulées. Le danger de l'alpha-cyperméthrine pour les invertébrés aquatiques et les poissons tient à sa toxicité aiguë. Rien n'indique toutefois qu'une exposition prolongée entraîne des effets cumulatifs.

On ne dispose d'aucune donnée concernant les effets de l'alpha-cyperméthrine sur les microbes terricoles. Les bactéries présentes dans les effluents n'ont pas paru affectées par une concentration de 3 mg/litre en système fermé.

La toxicité de l'alpha-cyperméthrine pour certains carabides et les larves de neuroptères est relativement faible et elle ne présente guère de danger pour les stades pré-imaginaux des hyménoptères parasitoïdes. Des études menées sur des champs de grande superficie ou de petites parcelles ont montré que l'alpha-cyperméthrine était peu dangereuse pour les carabides et les staphylinides mais qu'elle présentait un risque relativement important pour les linyphiides. Les effets sur ces populations d'insectes se sont limités à une seule saison de croissance. En outre, l'alpha-cyperméthrine ne présente guère de risque pour les larves de syrphides mais n'est pas dénuée d'effets sur les coccinellides. Malgré tout, la dissipation rapide des résidus présents sur le feuillage permet à ces animaux de reconstituer rapidement leurs colonies.

L'épandage d'alpha-cyperméthrine n'a pas d'effets indésirables sur l'abondance relative des arthropodes entomophages. Son utilisation sur les céréales à petits grains n'entraînerait donc pas la réapparition des ravageurs ou le déclenchement d'infestations secondaires.

Des études de laboratoire ont montré que l'alpha-cyperméthrine était peu toxique pour les lombrics. Des vers placés pendant 14 jours dans un sol artificiel contenant ce composé à des concentrations allant jusqu'à 100 mg/kg, n'ont présenté aucune mortalité.

Des études de toxicité aiguë également effectuées en laboratoire ont montré que l'alpha-cyperméthrine était extrêmement toxique pour les abeilles. Administré par voie orale, un concentré émulsionnable d'alpha-cyperméthrine a donné une DL_{50} à 24 heures de 0,13 μg/abeille, la valeur correspondante pour l'administration topique étant de 0,03 μg/abeille (de produit technique) ou 0,11 μg/abeille (de concentré émulsionnable). La forte toxicité de l'alpha-cyperméthrine pour les abeilles ne s'est pas manifestée au cours des épreuves de plein champ, probablement du fait que le composé a un bref effet répulsif qui réduit le butinage et, par voie de conséquence, l'exposition des insectes.

On ne dispose d'aucune donnée sur la toxicité de l'alpha-cyperméthrine pour les oiseaux.

2. Conclusions

2.1 Population générale

Lorsque l'épandage de l'alpha-cyperméthrine s'effectue conformément aux règles de bonne pratique, son utilisation en agriculture n'expose guère la population générale à ce composé et il y a peu de danger pour elle.

2.2 Exposition professionnelle

Moyennant de bonnes méthodes de travail ainsi que des mesures d'hygiène et de sécurité, l'utilisation de l'alpha-cyperméthrine ne devrait pas présenter de danger pour les personnes qui y sont exposées de par leur profession. L'apparition de sensations au niveau de la face indique une contamination. Dans ces circonstances, il est bon de revoir les méthodes de travail.

2.3 Environnement

Aux doses d'emploi recommandées, il n'est guère probable que l'alpha-cyperméthrine puisse être libérée dans l'environnement à des concentrations écologiquement dangereuses. Elle est fortement toxique pour les arthropodes aquatiques, les poissons et les abeilles dans les conditions du laboratoire. On ne peut envisager la probabilité d'effets toxiques importants sur les invertébrés non visés et les poissons qu'en cas de déversement accidentel, d'épandage excessif ou d'erreur de manipulation.

3. Recommandations

- Il convient d'éviter la contamination des eaux superficielles par l'alpha-cyperméthrine.

- L'alpha-cyperméthrine se lie fortement aux particules. D'autres études écotoxicologiques sont à effectuer à propos des effets de l'alpha-cyperméthrine sur les organismes qui vivent dans les sédiments car il s'agit d'un aspect qui n'a guère retenu l'attention jusqu'ici.

- L'absorption dans les voies digestives de l'alpha-cyperméthrine est à étudier dans diverses conditions expérimentales.
- Il faudrait également étudier la destinée de l'alpha-cyperméthrine après application sur l'épiderme.

- Il faudrait obtenir des données supplémentaires sur la toxicité à long terme, la cancérogénicité et l'immunotoxicité de l'alpha-cyperméthrine.

RESUMEN Y EVALUACION; CONCLUSIONES Y RECOMENDACIONES

1. Resumen y evaluación

1.1 Identificación, uso, destino y niveles en el medio ambiente

La alfa-cipermetrina contiene más del 90% del par de enantiómeros con mayor actividad insecticida de los cuatro isómeros cis de la cipermetrina en mezcla racémica.

Se trata de un insecticida piretroide sumamente activo contra una gran variedad de plagas habituales en agricultura y ganadería. Existe como concentrado emulsionable, formulacion de volumen ultra-bajo, concentrado en suspensión y en mezcla con otros insecticidas.

El producto técnico es un polvo cristalino, con buena solubilidad en acetona, ciclohexanona y xileno, y con baja solubilidad en agua. Es estable en condiciones ácidas o neutras, pero se hidroliza a pH 12-13. Se descompone por encima de los 220 °C.

No se dispone de información acerca de los niveles de alfa-cipermetrina en el aire.

Es probable que la degradación de la alfa-cipermetrina en agua se deba a procesos fotoquímicos y biológicos. El agua superficial y subsuperficial de un estanque rociado con 15 g/ha de principio activo contenía el 5% y el 19% de la dosis aplicada un día después del rociamiento, y 0.1% y 2% siete días más tarde. A los 16 días de la aplicación se encontró en el sedimento alrededor del 5% de la dosis utilizada.

Es probable que la alfa-cipermetrina se adsorba con fuerza a las partículas del suelo. Un año después del tratamiento con 0.5 kg de principio activo por hectárea se encontraron en el suelo residuos inferiores a 0.1 mg/kg.

El coeficiente de reparto *n*-octanol/agua de la alfa-cipermetrina es 1.4×10^5 ($\log P_{oa} = 5.16$).

Las tasas de aplicación recomendadas de alfa-cipermetrina son inferiores a las de cipermetrina, porque la primera es biológicamente más activa. En consecuencia, los residuos en los cultivos son escasos, y utilizando las tasas de aplicación recomendadas estos residuos oscilan entre 0.05 y 1 mg/kg. Los residuos en peces siluroideos marinos tratados con dosis entre el 0.001 y el 0.05% p/p de principio activo eran de 0.3-30 mg/kg una semana después del almacenamiento, y de 0.22 a 4.0 mg/kg tras 15 semanas de almacenamiento.

1.2 Cinética y metabolismo

La alfa-cipermetrina administrada por vía oral a ratas se elimina por la orina como sulfato conjugado del ácido 3-(4-hidroxifenoxi) benzoico y en parte como compuesto inalterado por las heces. De una dosis oral única alrededor del 90% se elimina del cuerpo en un período de cuatro días, y el 78% en el primer día. Los residuos en los tejidos son escasos, excepto en el adiposo. La concentración en la grasa tres días después de una dosis oral única de 2 mg/kg fue de 0.4 mg/kg. La eliminación a partir de la grasa es bifásica: en la fase inicial tiene una vida media de 2.5 días y en la segunda de 17 a 26 días.

La alfa-cipermetrina se metaboliza mediante la ruptura de su enlace éster. En la rata, el alcohol fenoxibencílico de la molécula se hidroxila y se conjuga con sulfato, y el ácido ciclopropano-carboxílico también se conjuga (probablemente en forma de glucurónido) antes de la excreción urinaria. En estudios con microsomas hepáticos de ratas, conejos y seres humanos se ha demostrado que la hidrólisis en el ester y rutas oxidativas se dan en las tres especies, si bien la primera es la ruta predominante en las preparaciones hepáticas de conejo y de ser humano.

En el ser humano, el 43% de una dosis oral (0.25-0.75 mg) se excreta en la orina en un plazo de 24 h en forma de ácido *cis*-ciclopropano-carboxílico libre o conjugado. La excreción urinaria no aumentó tras la administración de 5 dosis diarias sucesivas.

En la lana de las ovejas se detectaron concentraciones altas (hasta 1156 mg/kg) de alfa-cipermetrina 14 días después de la aplicación por inmersión o por lavado. En la grasa subcutánea se encontraron niveles bajos (hasta 0.04 mg/kg). Después de tratar terneros a lo largo del dorso con 10 ml de una preparación al 1.6%, no se detectó alfa-cipermetrina en los músculos ni en el hígado. La máxima concentración en la grasa perirrenal durante un período de 14 días fue de 0.26 mg/kg.

Tras la aplicación de hasta 0.2 ml de principio activo a lo largo del dorso de vacas lecheras, se encontraron en la leche de tres en 15 animales tratados residuos de alfa-cipermetrina en concentraciones que oscilaban entre 0.003 y 0.005 mg/ml.

1.3 Efectos en mamíferos de laboratorio y en sistemas de prueba in vitro

En roedores, la toxicidad aguda oral de la alfa-cipermetrina es entre moderada y alta. Los valores de la DL_{50} en ratones y ratas son muy variables y dependen de la concentración del compuesto y del excipiente. A efectos prácticos, se considera representativo un valor de la DL_{50} de 80 mg/kg de peso corporal. Sin embargo, se han notificado valores más altos de DL_{50} aguda por vía oral. La exposición oral aguda produce síntomas clínicos relacionados con la actividad del sistema nervioso central.

Las aplicaciones cutáneas aisladas de alfa-cipermetrina a ratones y ratas en concentraciones de 100 y 500 mg/kg de peso corporal, respectivamente, no produjeron mortalidad ni síntomas de intoxicación. La exposición de ratas por inhalación durante 4 h a una concentración atmosférica de 400 mg/m^3 tampoco ocasionó mortalidad ni signos clínicos.

Se ha reportado que la alfa-cipermetrina de calidad técnica produce una irritación cutánea mínima en el conejo. Algunas de las preparaciones provocan irritación ocular grave. La alfa-cipermetrina de calidad técnica no produce sensibilización cutanea. En cobayos ocasionó la excitación de las terminaciones neuro-sensoriales de la piel.

La exposición breve de ratas a concentraciones de alfa-cipermetrina de hasta 200 mg/kg en dieta diaria durante 5 semanas o hasta 180 mg/kg en dieta diaria durante 13 semanas no produjo efectos tóxicos. Con dosis más elevadas, las ratas mostraron signos de intoxicación asociados a la patología del sistema nervioso, disminución del crecimiento o aumento del peso del hígado y los riñones. No se pusieron de manifiesto efectos hematológicos, bioquímicos o histopatológicos claros.

En un estudio de toxicidad oral en perros durante 13 semanas, la dosis más alta, de 270 mg/kg causó síntomas de intoxicación, pero todos los demás parámetros examinados (relativos a la hematología, bioquímica clínica, análisis de orina, peso de los órganos, anatomía patológica e histopatología) se mantuvieron inalterados. El nivel sin efectos observados (NOEL) fue de 90 mg/kg de dieta (equivalente a 2.25 mg/kg de peso corporal al día).

En un estudio de toxicidad oral en ratas se demostró que la alfa-cipermetrina induce neurotoxicidad a causa de alteraciones histopatológicas de los nervios tibial y ciático, degeneración axonal y aumento de la actividad de la beta-galactosidasa.

Se carece de datos sobre toxicidad a largo plazo, toxicidad en la reproducción, teratogenicidad e inmunotoxicidad.

Con los datos disponibles sobre la alfa-cipermetrina, se puede deducir que se trata de un compuesto no mutagénico en las pruebas con *Salmonella typhimurium*, *Escherichia coli* y *Saccaromyces cerevisiae*, y en las pruebas *in vivo* e *in vitro* con hepatocitos de rata, con respecto a la inducción de aberraciones cromosómicas y producción de lesiones en cadenas simples de ADN. No se observó aumento de las aberraciones cromosómicas en las células de médula ósea de rata.

Se carece de datos sobre la carcinogenicidad de la alfa-cipermetrina.

1.4 Efectos en el ser humano

La exposición de la población general a la alfa-cipermetrina es insignificante siempre que en su utilización se apliquen buenas prácticas agrícolas. Se comprobó que la exposición cutánea profesional de los trabajadores durante la mezcla/carga, el rociado y el lavado del equipo era de hasta 2.94 mg, 0.61 mg y 0.73 mg, respectivamente.

En un estudio de exposición a la alfa-cipermetrina durante la formulación, se evaluaron los niveles de exposición mediante el monitoreo personal y estático de las concentraciones atmosféricas y la medición de los metabolitos en la orina. Los niveles de exposición personal media del grupo durante los dos días de la formulación de los concentrados de calidad técnica fueron de 2.8 y 44.9 mg/m^3, mientras que la exposición personal media del grupo al material técnico el tercer día fue de 54.1 mg/m^3. No se detectaron metabolitos en la orina (límite de detección, 0.02 mg/litro). Durante la formulación se informó de reacciones cutáneas ligeras.

No se han comunicado casos de envenenamiento.

1.5 Efectos en otros organismos en el laboratorio y en el medio ambiente

El valor de la CE_{50} (crecimiento) en las 48 y 96 horas para el alga de agua dulce *Selenastrum capricornutum* es superior a 100 μg/litro.

La alfa-cipermetrina es muy tóxica para los invertebrados acuáticos. Los valores de la CE_{50} (inmovilización) a las 24 y 48 h para *Daphnia magna* son de 1.0 y 0.3 μg/litro, respectivamente, y el valor de la CL_{50} a las 24 h para *Gammarus pulex* es de 0.05 μg/litro. La alfa-cipermetrina es muy tóxica para varios grupos de artrópodos acuáticos, pero lo es menos para los moluscos. Se puede reducir la toxicidad a corto plazo del compuesto formulando el producto como suspensión con mayor cantidad de aceite. Aunque el arrastre del rociado puede producir efectos tóxicos en los invertebrados acuáticos, la desaparición rápida de la alfa-cipermetrina del agua facilita la recuperación.

La alfa-cipermetrina es muy tóxica para los peces. El valor de la CL_{50} a las 96 h oscila entre 0.7 y 350 μg/litro, segun la formulación. Las formulaciones de concentrados emulsionables son mucho más tóxicas que el concentrado en suspensión, el polvo humectable y las formulaciones microencapsuladas. El peligro del compuesto para los invertebrados acuáticos y los peces radica en su toxicidad aguda. No hay pruebas de que se produzcan efectos acumulativos debido a una exposición prolongada.

No se dispone de datos acerca de los efectos de la alfa-cipermetrina en los microorganismos del suelo. En un sistema cerrado, no se observaron efectos en las bacterias de aguas residuales con concentraciones de 3 mg/litro.

La toxicidad de la alfa-cipermetrina para determinados coleopteros carábidos y larvas de neurópteros es relativamente baja, y representa un peligro limitado en las fases preadultas de los himenópteros parasitoides. En estudios de campo en pequeñas parcelas y en gran escala se ha puesto de manifiesto que la alfa-cipermetrina es poco peligrosa para los coleopteros carábidos y estafilínidos, pero es un peligro relativamente grande para las arañas linifíidas. Los efectos sobre las poblaciones se limitaron a una sola temporada de crecimiento. Además, la alfa-cipermetrina es de bajo riesgo para las larvas de sírfidos, pero tiene efectos considerables en los coccinélidos. Sin embargo, la rápida desaparición de los residuos de las hojas permite a estos animales recolonizar en poco tiempo las zonas tratadas.

La utilización de alfa-cipermetrina en el campo no diminuye la abundancia relativa de entomófagos en las comunidades de artrópodos. Su utilización en cultivos de cereales de grano pequeño no iría acompañada de la "reaparición" de plagas o de infestaciones de plagas secundarias.

En las pruebas de laboratorio, la toxicidad de la alfa-cipermetrina para las lombrices de tierra es baja. No se registró mortalidad tras 14 días de exposición de las lombrices a concentraciones de hasta 100 mg/kg de suelo artificial.

En pruebas de toxicidad aguda en el laboratorio se observó que la alfa-cipermetrina es muy tóxica para las abejas. La administración oral de una solución concentrada emulsionable dio una DL_{50} a las 24 h de 0.13 μg/abeja, mientras que el valor correspondiente para la administración tópica fue de 0.03 μg/abeja (producto técnico) ó 0.11 μg/abeja (CE). La elevada toxicidad de la alfa-cipermetrina para las abejas no se manifestó claramente en los ensayos de campo, probablemente a causa del breve efecto repelente del producto, que hace disminuir la actividad libadora de las abejas y, por consiguiente, su exposición.

No se dispone de datos acerca de la toxicidad del alfa-cipermetrina para las aves.

2. Conclusiones

2.1 Población general

Cuando la alfa-cipermetrina se aplica correctamente, la exposición de la población general al producto es baja y probablemente no supone riesgos.

2.2 Exposición ocupacional

Con buenas prácticas de trabajo, medidas de higiene y precauciones de seguridad, es improbable que la alfa-cipermetrina suponga un peligro para las personas expuestas en forma laboral. La aparición de "sensaciones faciales" es un síntoma de exposición. En estas circunstancias se deben re-examinar las prácticas de trabajo.

2.3 Medio ambiente

Con las cantidades recomendadas para la aplicación es improbable que la alfa-cipermetrina alcance niveles de importancia ecológica. En condiciones de laboratorio es muy tóxica para los artrópodos acuáticos, los peces y las abejas. Hay cierta probabilidad de que se produzcan efectos tóxicos importantes en invertebrados a los que no está destinado y en peces en casos de derrame, rociado excesivo o mala utilización del producto.

3. Recomendaciones

- Se debe evitar la contaminación de aguas superficiales.

- La alfa-cipermetrina se une fuertemente a las partículas. Se deberían llevar a cabo nuevos estudios ecotoxicológicos sobre los efectos del compuesto en los microorganismos de los sedimentos, puesto que este aspecto parece haber recibido poca atención.

- Hay que investigar la absorción gastrointestinal de alfa-cipermetrina en distintas circunstancias.

- Se debe investigar el destino final de la alfa-cipermetrina aplicada por vía cutánea.

- Hay que obtener nueva información acerca de la toxicidad/carcinogenicidad a largo plazo y de la inmunotoxicidad de la alfa-cipermetrina.